Jefferson M. Fish

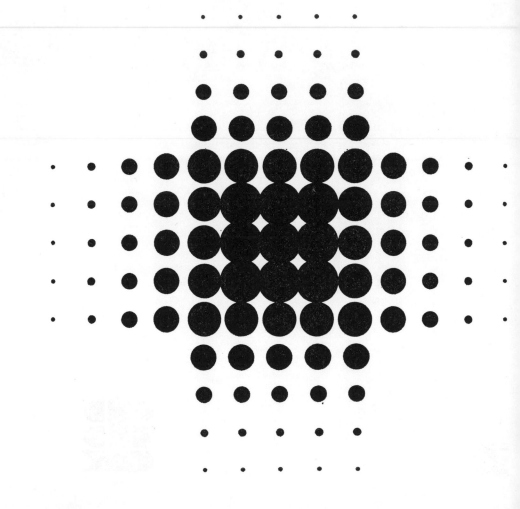

PLACEBO
THERAPY

Jossey-Bass Publishers

San Francisco • Washington • London • 1973

PLACEBO THERAPY
A Practical Guide to Social Influence in Psychotherapy
        by Jefferson M. Fish

Library of Congress Catalogue Card Number LC 73-9068

International Standard Book Number ISBN 0-87589-190-X

Manufactured in the United States of America

JACKET DESIGN BY WILLI BAUM

FIRST EDITION

Code 7332

The Jossey-Bass
Behavioral Science Series

Special Advisors

WILLIAM E. HENRY, *University of Chicago*

NEVITT SANFORD, *Wright Institute, Berkeley*

Preface

Physicians use the term *placebo* to refer to a substance which a patient believes will cure him of his malady—a belief that often proves justified—but which is chemically worthless. Such sugar pills have occasionally produced spectacular cures of otherwise untreatable illnesses. Because the drugs cannot be held responsible for these cures, the social influence process involved in administering them has been considered the active ingredient.

In this book I use the term *placebo therapy* in two related ways. First, it denotes a broad frame of reference for considering all forms of human interaction, especially psychotherapy, in terms of social influence processes. From this standpoint, the psychological elements involved in the medical placebo effect are a special case of much broader forces which affect virtually all aspects of our social existence.

Second, I use *placebo therapy* to refer to a method of

conducting psychotherapy based on social influence principles. Directive therapists, such as hypnotherapists and behavior modifiers, use specific techniques to ameliorate their patients' problems directly. Their approach is the opposite of the traditional, indirect one, in which therapists attempt to modify their patients' personalities in the hope that personality change will lead to a resolution of the patients' problems. For directive psychotherapists, placebo therapy is a set of principles governing all aspects of their therapeutic work except the content of the techniques they use. Controlled experimentation is the only means for discovering valid therapeutic techniques; placebo therapy is a strategy for getting the maximum therapeutic impact from such techniques, regardless of their validity.

In other words, placebo therapy is not another school of therapy. During recent years, many new kinds of therapy called by a variety of laudatory names have appeared. The various schools claim to be effective for scientific or philosophical reasons, and their adherents would be quick to assert that the titles are merely informative. Yet these new kinds of therapy are characterized by impressive though uninformative terms like *dynamic, intensive,* and *deep,* by terms bearing only a faint resemblance to their cognates in experimental psychology—*gestalt* and *eidetic*—or by terms similarly distant from their philosophical referents, such as *holistic* and *existential.* The proliferation of such schools of therapy, whose persuasive names are intended seriously, prompted me to call my creation placebo therapy, a nonschool of persuasion whose therapeutic title is intended ironically.

The purpose of *Placebo Therapy* is to convey a way of thinking and interacting clinically. In the course of discussion, I refer obliquely to many principles of clinical and social psychology, although I do not examine theoretical or empirical issues in detail. The Annotated Bibliography is for readers who wish to consider such issues at length.

In keeping with the clinical emphasis of this book,

illustrative case material relevant to placebo therapy is presented. The discussion of this material focuses on the therapist's strategy much more than on his patient's problems, and the interactions presented are meant to clarify particular issues, not to provide the most lifelike or elegant phrasing of the ideas involved. For example: Traditional therapist: "You seem to believe that some of the most important processes which take place in my therapy are unrelated to my theoretical orientation." "Placebo" therapist: "Exactly!"

Another use of such interactions or of statements by therapists is to illustrate the way a particular placebo might be delivered by the therapist. For example, "As you read this book, you will probably find some ideas which can be successfully applied to your own practice. Naturally, your first attempts at implementing placebo principles will be inexpert, so you may find only a few instances in which they are of help with your patients. Occasionally, your attempts may even backfire, but that is all right; such mistakes are part of the learning process. On the other hand, you may achieve dramatic success at the outset. In any event, as you gain more experience, you will be pleased with the impressive results you obtain."

This book is for Dolores and Krekamey.

New York City　　　　　　　　　　　　JEFFERSON M. FISH
September 1973

Contents

Placebo Therapy

*A Practical Guide
to Social Influence in Psychotherapy*

ONE

Psychotherapy and Faith Healing

Consider the following:

A depressed man who feels that he is worthless and that his life is empty goes to hear Billy Graham speak. Together with some others in the audience, he suddenly discovers God, sees a new meaning in life, and finds his entire existence transformed. Or, perhaps, he goes instead to a psychoanalyst's office, lies down on the couch, and gets up five years later, still depressed, with the "insight" that it was his mother who did him in.

What I want to know is this: Who is the better therapist? I think that the answer is painfully clear. Only a massive conspiracy on the part of mental health professionals could have maintained such an Emperor's New Clothes myth for so long. Just the idea of one man addressing a group of thousands, of whom hundreds step forth and probably dozens are deeply affected, provokes awe. That is group therapy! And the shame of it is that so few psychologists or psychiatrists have attempted to analyze the techniques of faith-healing and use them with their own clientele.

There are two possible explanations for why people like Billy Graham and Oral Roberts achieve such striking results. One is that the active ingredient in their treatment is God. That is their position, at any rate, and it is not one to be rejected lightly. Even medical men use the expression "I treat them; God cures them." Nevertheless, religion appears to have cornered the God market; and it is unlikely that psychology would have much success in attempting to compete.

The other possible explanation for the potency of faith-healing is that faith itself, and not God, is the curative agent. If so, then psychology can contribute much to the refinement and application of faith-healing. Psychologists could, for example, propose and test a social psychological model of how faith is awakened and applied therapeutically.

But why has this refinement not yet been done on a large scale? It is an acceptable practice for medical scientists to seek out faraway witch doctors and obtain the herbs they use to cure their patients. Scientists can maintain their respectability in such pursuits because they have the technology to distill the active medication, if any, from the sacred plants. The ritual in the context of which healing often takes place frequently goes unexamined, yet only the ritual is left when the herbs are discarded as medicinally neutral. Why, then, I repeat, are no psychotherapists paddling up the Amazon?

I can only speculate about this question, but my thoughts go to the heart of the thesis of this book. My guess

2

is that healing rituals in themselves have not been taken as seriously as healing herbs because herbs can be touched and behavior cannot. Surely behavior is just as real; after all, it can be *seen*. It is my guess that scientists are suspicious of things that cannot be touched and weighed and divided by two. I believe that willful ignoring of crucial phenomena such as faith explains why psychologists are not joining anthropologists in the field. Similarly, I think that the pseudoscientific trappings of mental health "treatments" enable practitioners to believe that psychotherapy is potent and that Oral Roberts is a fraud.

Despite the prevalent and comforting view that we are a rational people and that we save our faith for Sunday mornings, I find myself agreeing with theologians that our faith pervades every aspect of our lives. In fact, I can see no difference between the ways in which the lives of "primitive" peoples are governed by the "magical" beliefs of their cultures and the ways in which our lives are governed by the scientific beliefs of our advanced societies. The only difference is that science worship (or technology worship or individual-initiative worship) takes the place of voodoo in our world view. Ask the man in the street how he knows that the earth revolves around the sun, and you will see what I mean.

If faith is everywhere, it should follow that situations in which it is aroused abound in everyday life. The purpose of this book is to spell out ways in which faith can be aroused to ameliorate or cure psychological distress. A few examples from diverse social contexts illustrate my thinking.

The most straightforward example, and one with many parallels in psychotherapy, is that of a physician saying to his patient, "Take two aspirin for your headache." When the patient swallows the pills, two processes start. The first is that the analgesic effects of the pills, if any, take place; the second is that the placebo effects of the knowledge "This is aspirin" go to work. Although I do not wish to dispute the potency of such a scientifically blessed and highly profitable chemical as aspirin, I should point out that the dramatic effects of suggestion (that is, the placebo) on even severe pain have been thoroughly documented. In other words, it seems to me that the analgesic—at least in this case —is largely unnecessary. The longevity of Christian Scientists, whose faith is in things other than pills, attests to how many other drugs may be unnecessary.

But if a physician feels obliged to prescribe aspirin, a more desirable way to do so would be to remark off-handedly while writing the formula for aspirin on his prescription pad, "These are *quite* effective." Then, when the patient goes to the drugstore, he receives a medicine bottle, with the physician's name on the label, which states, "Take two for headache." Although some people may believe that aspirin is a powerful remedy, a procedure such as this would capitalize on the patient's faith in doctors, pills, and the healing ritual as it is practised in our culture.

When one begins to look at behavior from the point of view of faith-healing and similar placebo-induced modifications of expectations, he is able to identify such forces at work in unsuspected places. For example, when I was in Amsterdam a few years ago, I went to see the paintings in the Rijksmuseum. Like all other good tourists, I consulted my copy of *Europe on $5 a Day* and read that "Night Watch—which some acclaim as the greatest painting of all time—portrayed a number of these civilian-soldiers in shadows, obscured others entirely, cut off the bottom of one face with an outflung arm. The men of Captain Bonning Coq's troops were furious, and their enraged outcries caused all Amsterdam too look upon the portrait as a failure." When I entered the museum, I was immediately confronted by signs in several languages pointing the way to the Night Watch. As I walked through the museum, the periodic appearance of signs with arrows gave a mazelike quality to what was just a jumble of rooms. Finally I reached a huge gallery, where the massive painting was the only work on the far wall. Quite distant from the painting—too distant, I felt —chairs were arranged in an arc, as if they constituted a row in a theater. Nothing prevented one from getting near the painting, but a close-up view produced a surface glare which presumably was the reason for viewing the painting from a distance. The cameras and guidebooks identified most of the people in the room as tourists, like me. As I sat down, I heard one American ask another whether he was aware that the painting was once looked upon as a failure.

After participating in that aesthetic experience, I found myself convinced that any suitably sized old painting of a group of men could have been substituted for the original without changing the enraptured expressions of viewers. The guidebook publicity, the multilingual signs, and the theatrical display of the painting constituted a placebo so great as to make the painting itself almost irrelevant.

One other, related aspect of this artistic placebo deserves to be mentioned. The viewers of the painting were expected to be foreigners—as was evident from the guidebooks and signs. One would not expect the residents of Amsterdam to be equally dazzled by a painting in the museum down the block. Similarly, it is said that no native of Lourdes was ever cured at Lourdes; it is difficult to participate in a miracle at the shrine where one once played hopscotch. If a pilgrimage to a distant shrine is not in the family budget, the next-best way to be cured is to be on the spot when a distant healer comes to town. The appearance of Billy Graham in India or of the Maharishi in San Francisco is an occasion for lives to be transformed. In short, just as familiarity breeds contempt, so unfamiliarity breeds respect.

Respect for the source of the placebo is one of the most important ingredients in its effectiveness. In fact, some writers have been so impressed by the charismatic qualities of faith healers that they attribute the entirety of a cure to the patient's faith in the healer rather than to faith in what he says (this is what psychoanalysts mean by *transference cures*). Such an overemphasis ignores the fact that many placebos come from books, movies, television, and labels on medicine bottles. Nevertheless, respect for the source of a placebo—whether human or the written word—is an important ingredient in its effectiveness. Thus, when physicists say that man cannot fly and bicycle repairmen propose to build a flying machine, people naturally believe the former. Similarly, if a group of world-renowned astronomers were to assert that the earth has two hemispherical moons which merely look like a spherical orb when they are simultaneously visible, we would all modify our views of astronomy overnight. If a carpenter were to make the same assertion, he would be regarded as a lunatic.

We believe in our sources of information because they are usually correct. Similarly, the best placebo communications are true; truth cannot be contradicted, and the placebo therefore cannot be neutralized. One of the dangers in using placebo communications is that their recipient is vulnerable to counterplacebos. For example, in documented cases patients who were cured by new "wonder" drugs have relapsed when they heard that the drugs were ineffective. But if a drug is truly effective, a patient is not likely to worry that he got well to fast. In any event, the physician could say, "I'm glad to see that you're one of the people who respond rapidly to this drug."

I deal with the problem of phrasing placebo communications so that they are resistant to countercommunications in detail later. It should be mentioned in passing, however, that when faith healers attribute their cures to God, their "patients" cannot see, hear, smell, taste, or touch anything which could contradict this assertion. Such a position of power puts psychotherapists at a severe disadvantage. Only inspired maneuvers such as "You were cured by changes in the balance of forces in your unconscious" can rival such effectiveness, for it is the very fact that the patient is unaware of such changes which *proves* that the changes have taken place.

Thus, the processes which take place in psychotherapy are similar to those involved in curing in general and faith healing in particular. One might ask, therefore, why therapists do not refer their patients to faith healers. Although this is a complex question, I believe that the answer is primarily sociological. The clientele of therapists is different from that of faith healers. Billy Graham's converts are frequently healed well; therapeutic patients are predominantly well heeled. Furthermore, people who attend revival meetings usually already believe in God and hence are likely to be cured in a religious setting. In contrast, people who consult psychotherapists usually believe in psychology and are more likely to be cured in a psychological setting. Indeed, just as religious people find solace in their religion, the mass media are increasingly making it possible for outpatients to select therapists with congenial treatment philosophies. If a man wishes to unravel his castration complex so that he can ask his boss for a raise, he can do so directly by consulting a psychoanalyst. It is not necessary for him to undergo a conversion to a new belief system before being cured by an existential therapist.

Just as the best placebo communications are true, so it is highly desirable for the healer to believe deeply in his words because any doubts that he has may well be communicated nonverbally to his patient and thus subvert the cure. However, the faith of psychotherapists, particularly of believers in a given school, generally need not be questioned. A person usually studies to become a therapist only if he believes in psychotherapy. If he later loses his faith, the long and expensive years of training will all appear to have been wasted. In other words, his own belief functions as a solid protection against despair. In addition, psychothrapy is a lucrative profession. If a therapist loses his faith and quits practicing, he

7

loses the income; if he continues, he knows himself for a charlatan. Furthermore, personal therapy is a crucial part of a therapist's training. Such therapy is typically a long, expensive, and deeply involving emotional experience. Loss of one's faith inevitably negates this intense personal experience—and might well feel like a slap in the face to his therapist, who has subsequently become a colleague. Finally, if a psychotherapist does lose faith and it becomes public knowledge, he may also lose his sources of referral or even be punished for heresy by dismissal from his professional organization. In short, the consequences of a therapist's losing his faith are no less severe than those of a priest's losing his faith. It is not surprising that both are rare occurrences.

Perhaps this aspect of psychotherapy can be made clearer by a brief comparison of Sigmund Freud and Jesus Christ. Both were great healers who propounded revolutionary and heretical views of man. Both were dedicated men who gathered a group of disciples about them to spread the gospel. Both founded institutions dedicated to spreading their ideas, and each institution later fragmented into warring groups. Thus, within the superstructures of psychoanalysis and Christianity, the analyst and the priest can be seen to be in analogous positions. And while a Catholic priest and a Protestant minister may feel they have little in common, they share some basic assumptions which are so obvious to both of them as to remain unquestioned. In a similar way, psychoanalysts and client-centered therapists share almost no theoretical propositions concerning personality and psychotherapy. However, they do share assumptions about the institution of psychotherapy and the existence of an entity called personality which is changed by it. Moreover, these assumptions seem so obvious that neither group of therapists questions them. By drawing attention to the structural similarities between psychotherapy and religion, this comparison further emphasizes the role which faith plays in both.

Thus, the therapeutic transaction can be seen as taking place between two believers, the healer and the one to be healed, in something like the following form. Patient: "I'm sick." Therapist: "Participate in this healing ritual with me and you'll be well." (The patient then free associates or expresses affect or whatever he is supposed to.) Patient: "I'm well."

A few substitutions (for example, *sinful* for *sick*) make this outline appropriate for religious healing. Similar substitutions (*take this pill* for *participate in this ritual*) are appropriate for medicine. In any event, effective placebo therapy involves both the therapist's recognition of the context of therapy—the patient's "faith"—and his consequent choice of a ritual in which the patient can believe.

TWO

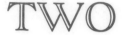

Overview of
Placebo Therapy

An overview of placebo therapy provides a framework for discussing the fine points of technique in later chapters. However, this overview is also critical to a proper understanding of the placebo approach because interventions are frequently so short-lived as to constitute an all-or-nothing form of treatment. For example, in a case of pain control, the therapist may want to structure his treatment so that it lasts for no more than a single session. In such a situation, the therapy session becomes a microcosm of an entire series of treatments, and the therapist has only one chance for his strategy to work. He is thus denied the luxury of thinking, "It isn't really essential for me to understand my patient at once since any mistakes I make can be corrected as new information emerges in subsequent sessions." Instead, he must integrate a limited amount of data with some principles of treatment and formulate a plan that has a good chance of succeeding.

The majority of cases do not involve such rapid treatment, and placebo communications serve more as an adjunct to other therapeutic techniques than as the primary method of treatment. Nevertheless, the statements which the therapist makes early in treatment frequently color the way in which all his later interventions—including placebo communications—are perceived. He should therefore have a clear picture of the entire course of therapy in order to communicate in a manner which has the greatest likelihood of ultimate success.

Figure 1 presents an outline of placebo therapy. This outline is intended as a practical aid to the therapist rather than as a theoretical model of psychotherapy. If the therapist thinks critically in terms of the areas and the sequence of processes diagramed in Figure 1, he will be able to apply placebo principles effectively. For example, the outline implies that the therapeutic contract is a major consideration in formulating a placebo; this idea is an important aid to the therapist.

The next three chapters cover the pretherapy, therapy, and posttherapy stages of treatment. The outline suggests both that the pretherapy stage is the most complex and that, once the placebo has been formulated, subsequent events should move smoothly in a sequential manner.

There are many reasons for the complexity of the pretherapy stage. Perhaps the most compelling is that the therapist must accurately predict his patient's response to the placebo communication. For example, if the therapist formulates a placebo which is not believable, the therapy stage will be a failure. If the placebo is believable but is too optimistic, complications will arise in the posttherapy stage.

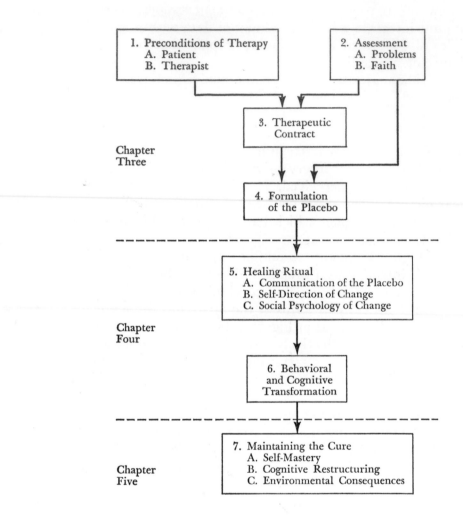

FIGURE 1.   Outline of placebo therapy.

Thus, if the patient expects to be cured but finds that his condition is only improved, he may well feel disappointed. This disappointment not only prevents further improvement but may even jeopardize the gains which have already been made. Therefore, in formulating a placebo, the following elements must be taken into account.

1. *Preconditions of Therapy.* Preconditions include not only the therapeutic setting but also thoughts about the setting on the part of both patient and therapist. The setting involves many questions for the therapist to consider. Does the therapy take place in the outpatient department of a hospital, in a clinic, or in private practice? Do people with power over the therapist have access to his records or have a different therapeutic orientation? Was the patient referred, or did he come on his own initiative? Do other people have a stake in his changing or in his remaining the same? Does the therapist have the primary responsibility for the patient, or is he only a consultant on a given problem? (For example, if the patient's analyst is referring him for pain control, it may be fine to alleviate his pain but catastrophic to interfere directly in his relationship with his wife.) What are the patient's assumptions about how therapy works and about the therapist as a person? What are the therapist's initial reactions to the patient? (If the therapist likes the patient very much and wants to do a lot for him, is there a danger of communicating an overly optimistic placebo? If he dislikes the patient, is there a likelihood of expressing this feeling? If the therapist feels that the case is nearly hopeless, is there a danger of communicating this negative expectation?) The answers to such questions are crucial if the therapist is to form a therapeutic contract which can be fulfilled. And, as discussed later, the therapeutic contract is one of the cornerstones of placebo therapy.

2. *Assessment.* During the process of assessment, the following kinds of questions arise: With what problems

13

does the patient seek help? If his complaints are vague, is it possible to discover specific problems through skillful interviewing? If the therapist cannot find any problems, is it possible to convince the patient that there is nothing wrong with him—or, failing this, to make up problems which he will agree are what "really" bother him?

Once the problem areas have been located, the therapist must formulate a believable placebo. To do so, he must assess the patient's strongly held beliefs or areas of faith. It should be stressed here that, to qualify as faith, a belief must be an integral part of a person's life. For example, some people who go to church regularly do so out of social motives rather than from religious conviction. Thus, the area of faith which could be used in therapy might involve the patient's need for friends or perhaps his social standing in the community, but not his faith in God. By contrast, a pantheist might well pursue a course of therapy which he believed would put him more in touch with the universal life force.

Usually, a belief in psychotherapy as a scientific procedure is sufficient for therapeutic purposes. However, regardless of the originality or banality of the patient's beliefs, the therapist must take care to understand them in order to formulate a helpful placebo.

3. *Therapeutic Contract.* Once the therapist has understood the preconditions of therapy and has assessed the patient's problems and beliefs, he is ready to form a therapeutic contract. This contract is not a legal document but a basis for a working relationship between patient and therapist in moving toward certain goals. The contract usually takes the form of a statement which appears ridiculously obvious to the patient, such as "If I understand what you've been saying, you'd like to feel more confident in social situations; and if you attain this confidence, you'll feel the ther-

apy has achieved its purpose." Once the patient approves such a statement, therapy can begin.

However, several points must be understood concerning the therapeutic contract. The therapist must remain open to the possibility of *not* contracting to do therapy with a particular person. If the therapist is personally opposed to the patient's goal or if the goal is unattainable, the therapist must refuse to proceed. Obviously, a therapist cannot work with a guilty thief who wishes to feel less guilty in order to leave fewer "absent-minded" clues. Similarly, a ninety-pound weakling who wishes to become a heavyweight champion should not be helped to get the courage to go into boxing. Naturally, if mortgage payments or a pregnant wife pressure a therapist into making an unrealizable contract, the resulting therapy will be a sham.

If the patient and therapist can agree on the goals of treatment (that is, if a contract is possible), the precise form of the contract should be determined by *therapeutic* rather than ethical considerations. Everything that transpires between the patient and the therapist must be judged according to its implications for the patient's welfare. The wording of the contract is no exception, even though it must be formulated within the context of the preconditions of therapy, where such matters as the therapist's fee are clearly aimed at the therapist's welfare, not the patient's. In this way, the therapeutic contract can be seen as a crucial element in psychotherapy since it communicates a powerful message: "You are not crazy. You merely have problems *A, B,* and *C.* Once we deal with *A, B,* and *C,* you will be cured."

If the patient accepts this communication—and he must in order to close the contract—therapy is already well on the road to completion. Some people, for example, have a number of trivial problems which could easily be ignored. However, they insist on torturing themselves with the unfounded notion that these problems are symptoms of some deep-seated illness—presumably a variety of mental leprosy. If such people can agree that their only therapeutic need is to deal effectively with the trivia, then even if their problems remain, they may find themselves feeling much better because, in making the therapeutic contract, they shift from the belief "I am basically crazy" to "I am basically sane." The contract itself serves as the placebo, and the patient's belief in psychotherapy enables him to change his belief about himself.

In other words, because the contract itself is part of the therapeutic process, it must be formulated in such a way as to help the patient. Some of the specific implications of this point of view are discussed further in the next chapter. It should be noted here, however, that this therapeutic orientation suggests that the contract is frequently not as contractual as it appears on the surface. For example, if a person seeks help with problem A but is afraid to ask for help with the more serious problem B, the therapist may well have to "contract" to cure problem A at the same time he is covertly helping the patient to deal with problem B.

4. *Formulation of the Placebo.* Once the above steps have been completed, the therapist has enough information with which to build an effective placebo communication. This communication is designed to activate one powerful set of the patient's beliefs (his faith) to change another set of his beliefs (*his problems*). Placebo therapy can thus be seen as a form of spiritual judo in which the therapist uses the power of the patient's own faith to force him to have a therapeutic "conversion" experience.

5. *Healing Ritual.* Once the therapist has formulated the placebo, he can begin the healing ritual. In its simplest form, the therapist presents this ritual in two parts: (1) If you do X, then (2) you will be cured. The first part of the ritual involves telling the patient (with a believable

rationale) something that he himself can do to conquer his problem. In this book, we are not concerned with the details of what the X might be; suffice it to say that, if what the patient does is actually helpful, so much the better. The important point is that the patient must be persuaded that it is what *he* does, not what the therapist does, which results in his being cured. This belief is crucial because it implies that the patient is the master of his behavior rather than its servant.

This is not the place to indulge in a debate about free will versus determinism and whether, when the patient does what he is told to do and believes what the therapist wishes him to believe, he is truly exercising his free will. People on both sides of the free will controversy agree that a person's *belief* that he has free will is an important determinant of his behavior. Thus, a therapist must encourage his patient to believe that he is curing himself, whether or not the therapist believes it.

If the patient undertakes to follow his therapist's self-help instructions, he finds himself under the influence of tremendous psychological forces, all of which push him in the direction of change. The patient's expectations of help tend to improve his condition. Then, his knowledge that he is receiving expert attention is likely to increase this improvement. His need to maintain his other areas of faith, which have been included in the rationale for the healing ritual, tends to force him in the direction of therapeutic change. This pressure is in turn increased by his realization that, if he does not change, the money, time, and effort devoted to therapy will all have been wasted.

6. *Behavioral and Cognitive Transformation.* Given these pressures, some change—often dramatic—almost always takes place, and the therapist can then use the improvement as proof that change is possible. This proof, in turn, increases the pressure for further change, and a positive cycle is begun which culminates in a realization of, or at

17

least significant progress toward, the goals of the therapeutic contract.

7. *Maintaining the Cure.* Once the cure has taken place, a number of forces tend to maintain it. One is the feeling of self-mastery which results from the patient's view that he himself has produced the change. Second, his awareness of his new level of functioning leads him to think of himself and the world in a new light. These new attitudes in turn make it unlikely that he will resume his old behavior. Finally—and this goes back to the pretherapy stage—the therapist should have arranged the therapeutic contract in such a way that the behavioral transformation which takes place will be warmly received within the patient's immediate environment. For example, if a man is depressed because his wife dislikes him, it is unlikely that any new-found joy will last very long. Thus, a contract to relieve his depression is doomed to ultimate failure. A contract to modify his relationship with his wife might well succeed, however, and if he then ceases to be depressed, his environment (that is, his wife) will reward his new behavior.

I have already pointed out that effective faith-healing is a process which takes place between two believers. Because the faith of these believers is so ingrained as to remain unquestioned, there is always the danger that attempts to focus attention on it may backfire. For example, if a therapist points out to a physicist the irrationality of his faith in a universe governed by physical laws, he may not respond with productive introspection. Rather, he may dismiss such a suggestion as incorrect or trivial, or he may misinterpret what is meant, or he may even regard the source of such enlightenment as a crackpot or a fool. The reasons for such reactions are evident. To function as a physicist, he has to believe in a universe whose nature can be uncovered by rational inquiry. However, since faith is irrational, the physicist must also deny, overlook, or otherwise deal with his

18

faith in order to appear rational to himself. Similarly, a book such as this, which emphasizes the irrational faith of patients and therapists alike, may have effects different from those intended. I am drawing attention to the omnipresence of faith in psychotherapy so that therapists can deliberately use their patients' faith to help them. If, after reading this book, a therapist attempts to contain or eliminate the role of faith in his psychotherapy rather than to use it as it already exists, my efforts will have been wasted. If a patient reads this book and uses it to keep his therapist from "putting one over on him" rather than to strengthen his belief in his therapist and what he says, placebo therapy will have become a self-defeating prophecy instead of a self-fulfilling one. Consequently, before spelling out the details of this approach, I am including the following admonitions in an attempt to forestall such misapplications.

Note to Patients. The thesis of this book is that if you believe deeply that you will be cured by what happens in your psychotherapy, then you probably will be cured. However, many people are hesitant to approach as new and unique an experience as psychotherapy with anything approximating a gullible frame of mind. They are mistaken in their implicit assumption that an "I'm from Missouri" attitude will not affect their treatment. Such apparent objectivity can only prevent faith from doing its work. Moreover, the stance of objectivity is based on the incorrect belief that psychotherapy is a rational process. Many different theories of psychotherapy generally agree that treatment is largely, if not exclusively, an irrational process. Among the irrational forces which have been deemed curative in psychotherapy are the patient's insight, recovered memories, and expression of feelings; the therapist's empathy, warmth, and genuineness, or inscrutability; the evocation or resolution (or both) of particular feelings of the patient toward the therapist; and a variety of conditioning procedures and chemical and electrical treatments. To these I add faith.

19

None of the above processes is rational. In fact, people usually go to a therapist only after all attempts at rational persuasion or reasonable advice have failed. When a patient says, "I know I shouldn't get so depressed when I'm criticized, but I can't help it," he is admitting that his problem is irrational. And, though he may have deduced the irrationality of his reaction on his own, a number of friends have quite likely told him, "Cheer up! It isn't so terrible to be criticized. No one can be right all the time." Similarly, a person who is terrified of dogs knows that there is no danger; and it is a waste of time to tell him, "This little dog can't hurt you." People simply do not consult psychologists for help with their fear of grizzly bears.

Psychotherapy heals irrational problems in an irrational way. The particular form which the irrational treatment takes depends upon the therapist's theory about the workings of irrational problems. *It is his theory, not his treatment, which is rational.* In this respect, treatment based on placebo principles is no different from that based on any other approach. Furthermore, the irrational faith which it requires from a patient is no more extreme than the irrational beliefs and fears for which he seeks help. A patient who says, "I believe that I am worthless, but I doubt that you can help me," really means, "I am willing to believe something irrational if it makes me miserable, but not if it makes me feel better."

You can choose between two irrational attitudes: "It seems as if this therapy should help me" and "Don't get your hopes up. Just wait and see what happens." You should suppress as unreasonable the second statement, not the first. The fact that you are in psychotherapy suggests that you harbor at least a germ of belief that it can help you—and it is in your best interest to nourish this belief rather than to deny it. If you find after a reasonable period that it is impossible for you to feel any change for the better or to believe that such a change is forthcoming, you should go to a different therapist. In any event, the nature and degree of your faith in psychotherapy are not matters to be taken lightly; such beliefs provide much of the power which will enable you to overcome your problems.

Note to Therapists. The purpose of this note is to warn against two misuses of placebo principles. The first, which involves practicing faith-healing with the wrong frame of mind, is potentially destructive; I refer to it as the con artist fallacy.

A therapist's first responsibility is his patient's welfare. Thus, when he says something to his patient because of the effect that it will have rather than because of its truth (that is, the therapist makes a placebo communication), he is acting in the highest therapeutic tradition. To be professionally responsible, such actions must not be self-aggrandizing. If the therapist uses the therapeutic situation as an opportunity to demonstrate his omnipotence, he is likely to distort the normal therapeutic contract—"I'll try to help you to cure yourself." "I'll try to be cured."—into something like the following. "I'm so much smarter than you that I can con you into being cured." "I'll try to be cured, . . . but you can't con me into anything." Such an approach would not prove therapeutic because the appropriate response to a con artist is a refusal to be conned. Moreover, not only is such an affirmation of the therapist's brilliance irrelevant to the patient's welfare, but the competition disrupts the harmonious work toward a mutually agreeable goal.

Because therapy takes place between two believers, a therapist who believes in placebo principles need never be guilty of being a con artist. He not only realizes that the placebo communication must be in his patient's best interest but also believes that the patient's faith, not his own brilliance, is responsible for the cure. Such a therapist need not worry that he will communicate the smile of one-upsmanship.

The second misuse of placebo principles, which involves half-hearted faith healing, I refer to as the dilettante fallacy. Many excellent clinicians eschew allegiance to a single school of therapy and continually experiment with new techniques and approaches. This orientation suggests a laudable openness to improving their work; and one of the goals of this book is to encourage such experimentation. However, these clinicians frequently display the sort of scientific attitude consonant with their innovativeness. When such a therapist tries a new technique, he wants to evaluate its effectiveness. An evaluation is certainly in order if he is to function responsibly, but from the standpoint of this book, he must not communicate to his patient that he is waiting to see whether his placebo statement works. The way in which the statement is communicated is an important part of the treatment. One cannot expect half an appendectomy to cure appendicitis; and a placebo statement which is made with less than full confidence will be similarly ineffective. It cannot be overemphasized that therapy takes place between two believers.

"In that case," an innovative therapist might ask, "how can I give your ideas a fair trial if I do not yet believe in them?" To answer this question, it is necessary to distinguish among three elements: the truth of the placebo communication, the therapist's belief in the truth of the placebo communication, and the therapist's belief in the curing power of the placebo communication. It has already been pointed out that the first element is desirable—though by no means necessary—for effective therapy. As for the second element, it should be clear by now that it is the therapist's duty to act as if he believes in the truth of what he says. Although this stance surely increases the therapeutic power of any lies he finds himself forced to tell, it unfortunately has the paradoxical effect of diminishing the potency of any true statements he makes because he realizes that the truth of his statements is independent of their healing power. In other words, as a result of denying his belief in science ("truth cures") and replacing it with a belief in placebo ("faith cures"), the therapist may nonverbally communicate his belief that it is unimportant whether his statements are true. Unfortunately, such a communication may be disruptive because the patient must believe in the truth of what his therapist says. Given the leveling effect of the therapist's relative indifference to the truth of what he says, the weight of the nonverbal communication must therefore be carried by the third element, the therapist's belief in faith healing.

Let us briefly reconsider the example of the physician whose patient has a headache and who writes a prescription for aspirin while remarking, "These are *quite* effective." His words and actions strongly imply both that the pills will cure the headache and that he believes the pills will cure the headache. There is no scientific basis for his asserting beforehand that the pills will work, and, as mentioned, his belief in such an assertion is more or less irrelevant. It is his belief in the healing power of the placebo communication which is responsible for his apparent confidence. Thus, a therapist who believes in placebo principles can remain relatively confident that his nonverbal communications are therapeutic; the therapist who is experimenting with a new approach does not have the same advantage. He must act not only as if he believes that what he says is true, but also as if he believes that the communication will have a therapeutic effect.

If the therapist does act as if he holds these two beliefs, then he is giving this approach a chance. Naturally, if he succeeds, the second *as if* will likely gradually become a firm belief in the power of faith. But if the therapist does not make a sincere effort to appear credible to his patients in these ways, his placebo communications are unlikely to have any perceptible effect. And then he would have no more right to expect a cure than a dilettante would have a right to expect his sketches to hang in the Rijksmuseum.

THREE

Preparing the Placebo

In placebo therapy, therapeutic transactions start at the beginning of the first session. The therapist's first statement to his patient may be a therapeutic maneuver—reassurance, for example. As pointed out earlier, the contract itself may be part of the therapy. Indeed, any aspect of any treatment stage may have a therapeutic impact. The processes outlined in Figure 1 therefore overlap; they were isolated more to permit conceptual clarity than to show them as distinct elements in an exact time sequence. However, the first four parts of the outline roughly constitute the pretherapy phase of placebo therapy.

When a patient first walks into a therapist's office, the most important information about the patient is that he is there. His presence implies that he is suffering in some way and that he has come to undergo the ritual which will make him well. The need for this ritual suggests that a person may get locked into a "mentally ill" role which is difficult to shed without help. If a therapist is shrewd enough to identify such a situation at the outset, he may be able to shorten the length of treatment considerably. A parallel is the old story of a man who went to a gym with his friend to play basketball. While they were undressing in the locker room, he saw that his friend was wearing a woman's panties. "Since when have you been wearing those?" he asked in amazement. "Ever since my wife found them in the glove compartment of our car!" his friend replied.

Someone in a similar situation might well consult a therapist for help with his transvestism. After a single session, the man would be able to announce to his wife that the insight he had gained relieved him of the need to wear a woman's panties. Of course, if he were too guilt-ridden to admit to his ruse and preferred to focus on other causes (for example, "I get anxious when I'm not wearing them"—an appropriate fear of getting caught), a different strategy would be necessary.

For example, the therapist might tell him that hypnosis has been found to be an effective cure for transvestism. If the man agreed to try this cure, the therapist (with the man present) might telephone his wife and warn her not to be startled if he returns home cured after one session. Then a dramatic hypnotic induction and the suggestion "once you open your eyes, you will no longer need to wear a woman's panties" should be sufficient to cure him. The therapist might equally well choose to teach the man self-hypnosis and allow him to cure himself. In either case the hypnotic ritual gives him a face-saving way to escape from the mentally ill role.

The purpose of this illustration is not to highlight different therapeutic strategies but to show the way in which the preconditions of therapy can be used in planning the therapy. In this case an alert therapist perceives that the goal of therapy is to get the man off the hook with his wife and thereby permit him to stop wearing panties. The therapist's socially sanctioned role of healer enables him to effect the cure; a baker or a dentist could not perform the same one-session miracle.

My recent work with a man in a clinic setting shows the importance of eliciting information relevant to the preconditions of therapy. He was in the process of getting a divorce, and his wife was seeing one of my colleagues. Because my client was clearly uncertain about whether he could have faith in me and the services offered by the clinic, we devoted more than half of the first session to a discussion of confidentiality, the possibility of my talking with his wife's therapist, the sorts of help that I could and could not offer, fees, scheduling of appointments, and similar issues. Only after we were satisfied that we understood each other concerning the preconditions of therapy did I ask him why he was seeking help. I am convinced that this discussion enabled him to be frank in stating his problems, and we were able to reach a contract within the remaining fifteen or twenty minutes of the session. If I had ignored his uncertainty, I believe that the first session would have been wasted in a fruitless attempt to get him to be specific about vague complaints. Moreover, if I had explored his hesitancy to open up in a manner implying that it was a symptom ("why are you so paranoid?—or insecure?—or resistant?"), I would have launched therapy with a negative communication, which would inevitably have encouraged his self-doubt and made him feel worse.

Just as the therapist must elicit information relevant to the preconditions of therapy, he must carefully explore the patient's problem areas and beliefs. These requirements force the therapist to focus more on information and facts than on other approaches. For example, because the healing ritual involves telling the patient exactly how to handle a particular problem, the therapist must know exactly how the patient is currently handling the problem; only in this way can he tell him what to do differently. Only a skilled interviewer can elicit such material at all—let alone smoothly—and therapists who are used to focusing exclusively on feelings are likely to experience considerable discomfort when they first attempt to modify their interviewing style.

Because the therapist must obtain particular kinds of information in order to plan his placebo, he must be careful not to fall into the trap of simply asking specific questions about what he needs to know. Though such questions are sometimes appropriate, they frequently structure the therapist-patient relationship into something other than a healing one. The poker-faced therapist who bombards a patient with questions about masturbation, extramarital sex, suicidal thoughts, and hallucinations, pausing only to write an occasional note on the pad in his lap, may well appear more like a DA than a DR.

Instead of taking such an oversimplified approach to eliciting specific information, the therapist must use at least as much interviewing skill and sensitivity as is necessary in exploring feelings. One way to do so is to be as specific as possible and encourage the patient to do the same. Thus, depending on what the therapist wants to hear more about, either "you wanted to see *Hamlet* that night" or "you wanted to go out with Ann" is preferable to "you wanted to go out that night."

Another principle to bear in mind is that the answer to "what did you do then?" is as important as the answer to "how did you feel then?"; the world responds to one's actions (including nonverbal actions), not to one's feelings. If a therapist can find out what his patient does, he may be able to find out why, for example, his patient believes that

27

the world treats him unjustly. Even though people's actual behavior occasionally bears only a remote resemblance to what they say they do, they are usually capable of reasonably accurate self-descriptions.

Many therapists discourage discussions of the specific details of their patients' behavior because they may concentrate on such material to avoid the anxiety involved in talking about feelings. However, sophisticated patients can also engage in phony self-exploration to avoid the embarrassment of admitting how they acted in a difficult situation. Furthermore, some people's speech is so abstract that they have trouble coming to grips with a specific question. Whatever the reason for a patient's evasiveness, the therapist must make every effort to gain the information he needs. One way to do so is to keep bringing the patient back to the question at hand. Each time the therapist reiterates his question, the pressure on the patient to respond is greater, and the therapist should soon be able either to get the information or to see that it is impossible to do so.

An alert clinician not only can get an answer to his question but also can assess both the reason for the difficulty in answering and how much help is required to remedy it. Consider, for example, the following conversation. Therapist: "How much did the car cost?" Patient: "I think I got a good price. I went to several dealers, and this was the cheapest. Of course, it has a clock I don't need, but even so, I think I did pretty well." Therapist: "I'm sure you did, but how much did it cost?" Patient: "Well, it's early in the year, so prices are on the high side. But it's still under the three thousand dollars I set as my maximum." Therapist (laughing): "How many dollars did you pay for the car?" Patient: "Twenty-nine hundred." The therapist has to ask the question three times to receive an answer. The patient's evasiveness appears to result from his need for the therapist's approval of his competence in buying a car, but he is capable of giving a direct answer when forced to do so. The therapist's comment, "I'm sure you did," and his laughter (as opposed to repeating the question with annoyance) show consideration for the patient's need for approval. At the same time, the therapist's persistence results in his obtaining the information he wants.

The process of gathering specific relevant information enhances the patient's view of the therapist as a scientific healer. This process implies to the patient, "Once I know what is wrong with you, I can cure you." Unfortunately, some well-read patients think that free association or the therapeutic relationship is responsible for change. Such people are naturally upset at the therapist's wasting time by asking questions when he should be relating. In these cases a comment such as "this is part of the diagnostic stage" or "yes, some therapists do work that way" conveys the reassuring information that the therapist knows what he is doing and that focusing on areas other than feelings is permissible.

The way a therapist handles the relationship with his patients stems in large part from his theoretical orientation. Orthodox Freudian analysts believe that, if they say very little and provide little information about themselves, their patients' reactions to them will exemplify feelings appropriate to significant people in the patients' lives. That is, the reactions are to mental representations (or *imagos*) of people (especially parents) as they were perceived by the patients (especially in their childhood). In contrast, Rogerian therapists believe that, by communicating feelings of non-possessive love (that is, Unconditional Positive Regard), they create a climate in which their patients can grow. If a therapist changes his orientation from Rogerian to psychoanalytic, his behavior can be expected to change accordingly. In other words, a therapist acts with his patients in a manner more or less consistent with his theoretical view of psychotherapy. I would like to place special emphasis on the word *acts*. I do not mean to imply that a therapist is phony in his behavior—phonies do not inspire the confidence necessary to effect a cure—but merely that the therapist assumes a particular role vis-à-vis his patient. Just as there is great room for individual variation in enacting the role of teacher (or father, or secretary, or mental patient), so there is plenty of opportunity for a person to "be himself" in the role of psychoanalyst. However, as a socially sanctioned healer, a therapist must conform to the demands of his role because he is dedicated to the welfare of his patients. Thus, if he believes that expressing love will cure his patients, he is ethically bound to express it.

The therapist's role in placebo therapy involves acting in ways which inspire faith because he believes that the patient's faith cures him. However, therapists vary in their ability to inspire faith, just as patients vary in their ability to be inspired.

In my experience few therapists have the charisma necessary to be an evangelical faith healer. Most tend to be reserved and introspective. Although an Oral Roberts may dwell within the heart of each Walter Mitty therapist, most therapists evoke a quiet faith in their professional competence rather than the frenzied devotion typical of revival meetings. Of course, each therapist is an individual whose manner inspires faith in some respects and doubt in others. A therapist must therefore assess his impact on patients so that he can accentuate the positive and eliminate (or modify or conceal) the negative. The comments of his supervisors, colleagues, and patients can be useful here.

Just as therapists differ in both the ways in which and the degree to which they can inspire faith, patients differ in the ways in which and degree to which they can be inspired. Consider, for example, the impact of a therapist's dress and of the decor of his office. If the therapist is in private practice and his clientele consists mainly of businessmen

30

and their wives, a business suit and a professionally deco-
rated office probably would inspire the greatest confidence.
If, however, the therapist works in a clinic serving mostly
hippies, such attire and decor would constitute a major barrier to the healing process. Although the therapist cannot
change his dress or his office for each patient, he can change
the way in which he relates to each patient in a manner
designed to use the patient's beliefs, needs, and expectations
in furthering the therapeutic goals. For instance, professors
are usually more formal than students, and a therapist can
inspire more faith in members of both groups if he adjusts
his speech and manner accordingly.

The issue of the degree to which patients are capable
of being inspired is a complex one and is discussed further
in Chapter Six. Suffice it to say here that psychologists have
discovered that, under standard conditions, people differ
consistently in their degree of suggestibility (or hypnotizability). The implication of this discovery for placebo therapy is that, once a therapist has assessed his patient's degree
of suggestibility, he can formulate his placebo communication in the most effective way. If his patient is extremely
suggestible, the therapist can say, "Your problem seems to
be X, and if you do Y, you'll be cured." If, on the other
hand, his patient is only slightly suggestible, he must give a
much more elaborate explanation, encourage questions, give
persuasive answers, and generally go to greater lengths to
get his message across.

In summary, probably the most distinctive aspect of
the therapist-patient relationship in placebo therapy is the
therapist's attitude during the interview. This attitude involves great sensitivity to the impact of his words on his patients—especially the impact on their interpretations of the
healing process. For example, a therapist should be able to
judge whether, if he should say, "I can help you," his patient
would view him as a savior or a fool. Once a therapist

acquires this skill, he finds that the rest of the therapy becomes much easier. Although outwardly his interviews may seem relatively unchanged, a therapist working in this way says things for the effect they will have rather than for his belief that they are true. Thus, instead of speaking empathically because he believes that empathy cures, he does so because he sees that such statements add to his credibility in his patient's eyes. Furthermore, once his patient feels understood, the therapist can on occasion take the liberty of distorting his empathy for a therapeutic reason. Instead of saying, "You feel worthless because she left you," he might say, "I sense a reluctance on your part to admit that you also feel relieved that she's gone." Of course, such distortions must be used sparingly and must bear directly on the goals of therapy. From a social influence viewpoint, however, such distortions (as well as truly empathic statements) should be judged in terms of their therapeutic effect rather than in terms of their truth.

The therapist must also phrase the contract in a way that will have the greatest therapeutic effect. Although there are many ways to do so, the most obvious one is to formulate the contract in a way that inspires hope by defining clear-cut goals, communicating that the goals are attainable, and reassuring the patient that he is not crazy. The contract can also be phrased to anticipate possible future difficulties. For example, if the patient later hesitates to follow some of the therapist's suggestions, he can remind the patient of the therapeutic contract and use it to motivate him to work toward the agreed-upon goals.

Although this approach often speeds up the healing process, nothing is lost if the patient still refuses to cooperate because the contract contains an unwritten escape clause: Intermediate goals can be set up, the healing ritual can be changed, and if necessary the contract can be renegotiated. The therapist can say, "Though we could have saved some time if X had worked, it's clear that we should now do Y because of Z. Candidly admitting failure while offering an alternative may even increase the therapist's credibility because his patient may see the admission of failure as admirable honesty. Such an interpretation may make him more willing to accept the proposed alternative. Furthermore, even though they have failed to reach the goal, the therapist has had time to learn more about his patient and can use his knowledge to devise rituals with a better chance of success. For example, if a patient has seemed distressed at the speed and directness of the therapist's suggestions, the therapist can say, "I think that at this point a more deliberate and indirect approach, such as the following, is in order." If the patient has instead been losing interest in a long, drawn-out series of activities, the therapist can say, "We are now ready to enter a new and direct phase of therapy."

The structure of the therapeutic contract thus tells therapist and patient alike both when the goals are being attained (which inspires more faith and consequently more healing) and when no progress is being made (which tells the therapist to do something different). When the therapist sees that a new contract is necessary, he can derive more information about his patient from the process of formulating it and correct possible flaws in his original view of the case. Such a case is briefly discussed in Chapter Four.

Just as the contract may be modified during therapy, another contract may be formulated after the goals are reached. Desirable goals sometimes become apparent to the therapist as he works with the patient, and, as the patient progresses, he sometimes discovers new problems he wants to work on. New goals are often formulated after the original ones have been achieved when therapy has been proceeding on the basis of an unstated agreement either to change or not to change problem areas outside the contract. Consider, for example, a shy man who makes a contract with his therapist to get dates. The therapist may decide that the man really wants to have sexual intercourse but is ashamed of his sexual desires and feels that this goal is unattainable. Therefore, the therapist overtly helps him to get dates while covertly arranging the dates to maximize the possibility of sexual intimacy. If in getting dates the man also has intercourse, therapy will be terminated. If he becomes capable of getting dates but remains a virgin, the therapist might then discuss with him the advisability of setting a further goal. His success in geting dates will likely enable him to deal with the sexual question more openly and transform the unstated understanding with his therapist into a new contract.

Unstated agreements not to change other areas often present a greater problem because the therapeutic ritual may depend for its success on demonstrating a lack of change elsewhere. For example, a college student who makes a contract with his therapist to improve his grades may really be saying, "I'm willing to do better in school if I don't have to give up fighting with my parents." The therapeutic ritual might be based on demonstrating to him that he can antagonize his parents just as much while getting good grades as while getting poor ones. Once the student has achieved his goal of better marks, the therapist may want to set a goal of having the student give up fighting with his parents. However, unless the therapist can find a more attractive substitute activity (having no contact at all with his parents, for example, or having a more fulfilling relationship with a member of the opposite sex), he may have to be content with terminating therapy after attaining only the goals of the initial contract.

The only therapeutic contract which cannot be changed is one including an agreement not to change it. Certain kinds of time-limited therapy, for example, depend for their effectiveness on an ironclad agreement that therapy will last no longer than a given number of sessions. The therapist cannot say at the end of the last session, "We're so near our goal that I'll see you for another session"; one purpose of limiting the number of sessions is to force patients to deal rapidly with unpleasant material; and extending therapy beyond the agreed-upon limit may make the patient feel that the original deadline was a deception on the part of the therapist.

However, even in time-limited therapy, the therapist does have a way of renegotiating the contract because the contract is between only the patient and him (and, perhaps, the clinic where he works). The therapist can say, "We have made this much progress in our ten sessions. I can't see you any longer, but I can refer you to Dr. X at the Y Agency, who can work with you on these other areas." Then, after obtaining a release form from the patient, the therapist can call Dr. X, discuss the case with him, and advise him about what sort of contract might be appropriate. Thus, even "unchangeable" therapeutic contracts can be renegotiated through the device of having another therapist carry out the new contract.

In summary, the therapeutic contract is an agreement which is in effect only as long as it has not been changed. Although the contract provides a useful structure for the conduct of therapy, the therapist should be ready to change it as soon as a different contract appears to be better suited to the patient's welfare.

No discussion of the therapeutic contract would be complete without a few observations about the fee—particularly that charged by therapists in private practice. Even a highly educated, very experienced, and widely published therapist is paralyzed with confusion when asked in public how much he charges for his time. Therapists' money anxiety makes therapy a transaction in which we cannot see the forest for the trees. We spend our time arguing over how deep (in inches?) we should make our interpretations and overlook the fact that the fee is the one area where we have our patients over a therapeutic barrel. After all, people enter therapy complaining of certain problems and must pay until they give up (are cured) and admit that the money bothers them more than their problems.

A therapist can get therapeutic mileage out of his patients' financial bind in a number of ways. If he structures therapy as a relatively short-term experience, his patients are more likely to count each dollar than during long-term treatment, and the sudden financial deprivation provides additional motivation to get well. In other words, short-term psychotherapy is likely to be viewed as an expensive brief experience (like adding a room to a house), while long-term psychotherapy comes to be seen as a fixed expense (like rent). A few therapists who have the courage of their convictions have recently reported success in making fee reductions contingent on improvement by their patients in specific areas, while other therapists secure postdated checks made out to their patients' favorite charities and mail the checks off if the patients do not make agreed-upon improvements on a week-to-week basis.

The patient who comes to a therapist for the first time arrives with several powerful motivations for change. He is probably acutely disturbed, which gives urgency to his need, and hopes to be helped in a miraculous way by the therapist's penetrating insight. He also is bothered by the probable cost of therapy, as well as by the feeling that his seeking help is proof that he cannot control his own behavior. Under these circumstances, an effective therapeutic communication, which maximizes all these motivations, goes something like this: "I can see that you are upset, and I think that I can help. I know that therapy will cost you some money, but if you're willing to work at dealing with your problems, you should be able to conquer them, or at least make significant progress, in a relatively short time."

The opening gambit of long-term therapists is almost exactly opposite: "I can see that you are upset and would like me to help you right away. Unfortunately, however, your difficulties are merely symptoms of an underlying personality problem, and they will not change until you gain enough self-understanding to resolve the personality problem. This process usually takes several years. I should mention that psychotherapy is a kind of joint exploration, so I cannot guarantee where our investigation will lead us or what its results will be. In other words, it may well alleviate the symptoms bothering you, but it also may not. My fee is thirty dollars per session, and I think that we should begin by meeting twice a week."

This sort of communication has at least as powerful an effect on the patient's expectations as the one I propose, but the effect is in the opposite direction. It demolishes the patient's hopes for a quick cure and forces him to accept the idea of living with his problems for a long time to come. The only virtue—if it can be called that—of such a communication is that it speeds up the process of socializing the patient to a new mode of existence: life with therapy.

One of the goals of therapy should be to make therapy unnecessary as rapidly as possible. Once therapy becomes a way of life, it is much more difficult for the participants to extricate themselves; the patient must give up a continual source of support and understanding, and the therapist must give up a fixed percentage of his income. After the patient has been in therapy for several years, he may throw good money (as well as time, effort, and emotional involvement) after bad in the hope that the resolution of his Oedipus complex is just around the corner. I know one man who stayed in therapy with the same therapist for ten years, and neither the patient nor his friends could see that any change had taken place. He spent the last five years in therapy in the hope that the first five (and then six and then seven . . .) would not have been wasted. When someone tells his friends, "I've already been in therapy for six years, and I'm determined to see it through," he is probably trapped in the same situation.

Let us now briefly consider the fee from the therapist's point of view. Facile explanations for the size of a therapist's fee range from his competence and his years of training to the desirability of charging a lot so that his patients will feel that therapy is important. Another explanation, which many patients are perceptive enough to sense, is that a therapist sets his fee at a level enabling him to live in the style to which he would like to become accustomed. Because the supply of therapists is small and the demand is great, achieving this goal is frequently possible.

A second, relatively minor, consideration is that a therapist may set a high fee to discourage people without problems from wasting his time. For example, I know of a clinic which offered free therapy for children. A suburban housewife, whose days included a fair amount of free time and boredom, brought her son in to inquire whether his left-handedness had any psychological significance. Needless to say, the psychologist who saw the woman was annoyed at having to waste a session and do the paperwork involved in opening and closing the file. He suggested that, if the woman had had to pay even one dollar for the session, she might have kept her curiosity to herself. (Incidentally, this example provides a good argument for clinics' charging fees on a sliding scale based on the patient's ability to pay. They might not charge any fee at the lower end; in our society a poor person who seeks help at a clinic is likely to have problems.)

A more important determinant of the fee is the social comparison process, in which the therapist matches his fee against those of his colleagues. Given the taboo on discussing money, this process is slow and imperfect, but, by talking with therapists who are close friends and with patients who

were treated by other therapists, a clinician in private practice can develop a general idea of current market conditions.
His fees are then determined by a desire to charge neither
too little (lest he appear incompetent or, perhaps, unconfi-
dent) nor too much (lest he appear avaricious).

In summary, then, the fee has great therapeutic potential. Unfortunately, therapists' anxiety about money and
the determination of the fee by exclusively extratherapeutic
considerations have prevented this potential from being
realized.

I have included these comments on the fee not only
because of their relevance to the implementation of placebo
principles but also because they illustrate an uncomfortable
kind of intellectual honesty which I feel therapists should
adopt. Another example is my statement that lying to a patient is desirable if the lie furthers the therapeutic goals, is
unlikely to be discovered (and hence backfire), and is likely
to be more effective than any other strategy. A therapist who
is strong enough to lie knowingly under these conditions is
likely to be more truthful in general with his patients than
one who self-righteously (and unreflectively) declares that
a therapist should never lie. Unilaterally applying such
moral imperatives to something as complex as life's problems is bound to be strained at times. For example, at the
end of an initial interview with an extermely hopeless and
lost woman who was planning to kill herself, I looked in-
tently into her eyes and said, "I can help you." If this statement was not a lie, it stretched the truth considerably; I believed that she was sincere about killing herself, and I was
not at all sure that I could help her. However, after speaking with her, I had concluded that she was under great environmental stress and that, if she could get through the
next few days, she would be out of danger. Thus, in addition
to making a few suggestions for reducing the pressures she
was under, I used one of the least subtle placebo communica-

tions as a means of giving her some hope for the immediate future.[1]

The same intellectual honesty enabling a therapist to lie under a particular set of circumstances is also responsible for his not deceiving both his patients and himself with such ridiculous pronouncements as "a higher fee makes patients value therapy more." This honesty with himself complements a therapist's sensitivity to the impact of his words. Since everything he says to his patient has an effect, it is a therapist's responsibilty to make that effect therapeutic.

Another, even less comfortable way of viewing this situation is that a therapist does not have the option of choosing whether or not to manipulate. He can only manipulate deliberately toward the therapeutic goals or manipulate blindly in undetermined directions. Given these difficult alternatives, I would certainly choose the former.

Even if he is equipped with both a sensitivity to the impact of his words and actions, and a willingness to communicate in ways which will further the therapeutic goals, the therapist must still decide on what message he wishes to communicate. Because the processes outlined in Figure 1 overlap, specifying how to formulate placebos is difficult. Any particular placebo communication must be based on the particular preconditions of therapy, the particular assessment of problems and beliefs, and the particular therapeutic contract of that particular case. Similarly, the problem of formulating a placebo is intimately bound up with the problem of devising a healing ritual for a given patient. Although the examples provided throughout the book give a more specific understanding of these processes, a few general comments can be made about the issues involved in formulating a placebo.

---

[1] She did not attempt suicide. Of course, I cannot prove that another approach or no therapy at all would have led to a different result. Because of the obvious risk in using an untreated suicidal control group, data on such situations are difficult to obtain.

From the patient's point of view, the initial phase of therapy appears to take place in a logical manner. He begins by telling the therapist why he is seeking help. Then the therapist encourages him to go into greater detail about his problems and related aspects of his life. Finally, the two agree on the goals of therapy and the fee and scheduling of appointments, and therapy begins. The therapist views this process differently. He makes the process appear logical to encourage the patient's faith in his therapist's competence and to confirm his expectation of being helped, but the sequence of the therapist's thoughts anticipates and is often the reverse of the sequence of events in the session. Generally, he first devises a healing ritual with a good chance of success, then develops a strategy for explaining the ritual in the most persuasive way, and, finally, outlines the goals of therapy in a manner that suggests the healing ritual and is consistent with the patient's beliefs and formulation of his problems. The therapist then reverses the sequence with the patient: He discusses the goals of therapy (forms a contract), explains the therapeutic strategy (communicates the most important placebo), and implements the strategy (continues with the healing ritual). Thus, the therapeutic strategy appears to the patient to grow out of the goals set in the therapeutic contract, but the goals are selected because the therapist already has good idea of how to go about reaching them.

In deciding on a therapeutic ritual, the therapist must consider both the actual validity of the ritual (the treatment effect) and the persuasive value of the ritual (the placebo effect). Although I concentrate on the latter, I do not want to imply that no ritual has any therapeutic validity. Different healing techniques, like different placebo communications, probably vary from quite helpful to quite harmful, depending on the individual patient and his particular problem. However, the validity of a given ritual is relevant here only insofar as it increases the patient's faith.

41

The persuasive value of a ritual, whether or not it is valid, stems from its intrinsic believability or its intriguing quality. A ritual clearly related to the goals of therapy is likely to be more believable than one which is not. Thus, if a person is seeking help for his fear of heights, suggesting that he climb stairs until he becomes anxious, rest until he is calm, and then resume climbing until he is again anxious constitutes a believable ritual. Telling him to sit on a park bench is not believable, but telling him to sit on a park bench and concentrate on the idea "the bench is safely on the ground, I am safely on the ground, buildings are safely on the ground; tall buildings cannot harm me" for longer and longer periods each day is believable. Both the fee and the necessity of spending several hours a day meditating on drivel would pressure the patient to give up his fear.

Intriguing or mysterious rituals can help patients who view therapy as a form of magic. Patients who have faith in science are more easily cured with a ritual which appears scientific, while those who are less self-conscious about believing in magic can be cured by magic. An intriguing ritual for a man with a fear of heights is to suggest that he see if he can detect any subtle differences among the shadows at 2 P.M. on window sills on the third, seventeenth, twenty-fourth, and forty-third floors of a particular building. If the suggestion is made in a confidential tone of voice—hinting that the patient may learn something important about his fear from the shadows—his curiosity may get him to the forty-third floor without anxiety. Realizing later that he was not anxious, the patient may discover that the shadows miraculously cured him.

In summary, preparing the placebo involves laying the groundwork for faith-healing to take place. The therapeutic contract identifies the problem areas and limits the patient's definition of his "mental illness" to a workable size. The patient's beliefs and the goals of therapy are then used to define clearly the "mental health" toward which he is aiming. Finally, the therapist devises a ritual (which may have independent therapeutic validity) and explains this ritual persuasively by phrasing it in terms of the patient's own beliefs.

FOUR

The Healing Ritual

Γhe middle phase of placebo therapy, which the patient sees as the therapeutic one, consists of three parts. First, the therapist explains the healing ritual persuasively, in terms of the patient's beliefs. Next, the patient undergoes self-cure. Finally, the process of self-cure allows the patient to shift from the mentally ill role to that of a psychologically unencumbered individual. I have already discussed the psychological rationale for this sequence of events, and this chapter presents illustrative material aimed at clarifying the ways in which the theory of placebo therapy is translated into practice.

Strictly speaking, this book is concerned with the persuasive value of the healing ritual in helping a patient with

44

his problems and not with the independent validity of the ritual itself. Furthermore, because the ritual should be tailored to the requirements of the patient, the number of possible rituals is as great as the number of people with psychological problems. Despite both these objections, however, the following brief descriptions are included to illustrate both the kind of thinking that goes into planning a healing ritual and the ways in which the placebo value of a ritual is intertwined with the independent validity of the ritual.

Placebo therapy emphasizes the use of one set of the patient's beliefs (his faith) to change another set of his beliefs (his problems). Thus, patients' faith in the truth of the information which comes from high-status sources, such as therapists and textbooks, provides the basis for a number of therapeutic maneuvers. In particular, such information can be used both to cure problems directly and to enhance patients' expectations of help from therapy.

One of the simplest healing rituals is persuading the patient that he has no problem. The arguments against the existence of a problem constitute the placebo communication, and obtaining such information from a prestigious source constitutes the healing ritual. It is the patient's belief in the truth of the information, rather than its actual truth, which is responsible for the cure. Thus, if a person believes that he has a deadly disease, he will feel anxious and depressed; and if he believes that the medication which he has taken has cured the disease, his emotional state will improve dramatically. This is the case whether or not he has such a disease, and whether or not the medication helps.

The following two brief examples illustrate the therapeutic value of providing information. In the first case, a young man expressed to his therapist his feelings of inadequacy concerning his "low sex drive." These feelings were based on the fact that he was unable to reach orgasm merely by having vivid sexual fantasies. The therapist assured him that he was misinformed and that it was impossible for any man to have an orgasm without tactile stimulation of his penis.

In the second case, a woman expressed concern to her therapist about her "frigidity." She explained that she had never experienced a vaginal orgasm but was limited to clitoral orgasms. *Human Sexual Response,* by William Masters and Virginia Johnson, had just been published, and the therapist suggested the woman consult that book to learn more about the female orgasm. Needless to say, the woman was astonished to find that the vaginal orgasm is a myth.

Although these two examples contain only a small part of the treatment of the two cases, they do shed light on a number of points. Clearly neither of the patients had a sexual problem (an abnormality of sexual performance). Rather, their difficulties centered around low self-esteem, especially their beliefs about the adequacy of their sexual performance. As they received new information from re- liable sources, their beliefs about themselves changed. The ritual in the second case involved self-cure because the woman discovered the information for herself. Furthermore, the discovery that her therapist possessed important scien- tific knowledge enhanced his credibility for future placebo communications. Finally, though the information given the patients appears to have been factually correct, it was their belief in the information—rather than its accuracy—which caused the improvement in their self-esteem. Thus, even if future research reveals that the vaginal orgasm does exist and that its discovery was hindered by a subtle methodolog- ical or sampling error, the improvment in the woman's self-esteem as a result of her new knowledge remains.

One of the strong points in the therapist's role as a socially sanctioned healer is his status as an expert on psy- chotherapy. Because of this status, patients frequently give their therapists considerable freedom in structuring their ex- pectations about their own therapy. Thus, most patients want to know what psychotherapy will be like; and they tend to be quite accepting when their therapists provide them with such "information."

Patients' beliefs that they are crazy usually constitute a major part of their difficulties; and their fears that they will not recover (that they are hopeless cases) are often a major barrier to treatment. If the healing ritual can be presented in such a way as to neutralize these beliefs and fears, patients can then be cured both to a greater degree and in less time than would otherwise be possible. The placebo communications used for this purpose can logically be divided into categories according to the point in therapy at which they are appropriate. Thus, some placebos initiate or lay the groundwork for change; some placebos suggest that the rate of change will accelerate; and some placebos defend against relapse. However, the form of all such communications is the same.

The placebo communication of defining everything as progress is based on the logical inference that, at any point in therapy, only three possible things can happen to the patient: He can get better, he can remain in the same condition, or he can get worse. By defining all three possibilities as progress, the therapist is able both to speed up therapy and to neutralize the patient's feeling that he is a hopeless case. Furthermore, by predicting all three therapeutic possibilities before the patient begins, the therapist can lay the groundwork for every conceivable placebo communication as therapy progresses. Thus, since therapy is supposed to be of help, the patient is encouraged in his belief that he will get better. As soon as he reports any improvement, his therapist can point out that therapy has begun to work and can suggest that the rate of improvement will accelerate. Similarly, the therapist can predict that sometimes progress may occur slowly. Then, if a patient reports that his condition is unchanged, the therapist can agree that his current level of progress is quite slow; but he can predict that as soon as the current stage of therapy has ended, the patient's rate of improvement will accelerate. Finally, a therapist can mention that, because of the nature of psychological problems, on rare occasions a patient may regress if he has reached a point where such regression enables him to learn to cope with his problems. If the patient gets worse, the therapist can sympathize with him over how painful progress can be, while suggesting that once he has benefited from his therapeutic regression, he will be able to make still greater and less painful strides. Such a statement can prevent the patient from feeling miserable about his misery—and thus increase the likelihood of a turnaround in his condition —but it would be disastrous for the therapist to believe such nonsense. Rather, any unexpected worsening of the patient's problems is a strong hint that the therapist's assessment is incorrect; it should be taken as a signal to begin the diagnostic process anew and reevaluate all assumptions about the case.

The strategy of defining all possibilities as progress ahead of time and then building on whatever happens can also be applied to the prevention of relapses after the patient leaves therapy. Thus, the therapist can, in the last session, make an explanation such as this to the patient: "Life has its up and downs. Of course, if you should develop any new problems which you cannot handle, you can always return to see me—although it is unlikely that you will need to do so. Rather, I think that you will be able to handle the difficult times when they occur and bounce back from them as well as other people." This communication has several virtues. It reduces the patient's feeling of being abandoned by the therapist because it reassures him that he can always return. It emphasizes his ability to function on his own. And, by defining any future difficulties as resulting from life's ups and downs, it guards against the patient's subsequently labeling himself as mentally ill and acting in accordance with that label.

An important healing ritual, which is associated primarily with behavior modification, involves having the patient approach his therapeutic goal in small, carefully defined steps, with the therapist providing considerable structure, information on his performance, and encouragement. The direct relevance of such a ritual to the patient's problem encourages his expectation of help. In addition, the small steps enable him to avoid the pessimism associated with failure, while his gradual successes contribute to his self-esteem. These placebo aspects of such a ritual can easily be seen to be bound up with any conditioning which takes place.[1]

    This healing ritual can be illustrated by my weekly meetings, at a university clinic, with an advanced graduate student in engineering. He was extremely shy and socially awkward, and he was seeking help to increase his currently nonexistent contact with women. At our first session I instructed him to make eye contact with and smile at every attractive woman he passed. We practiced his smiling at me and vice versa until he got the idea. At our second session we discussed his experiences of the preceding week, especially the minute details of how he had felt, how well he had been able to make eye contact, and how relaxed his facial expression and smile had been. Then I added the instruction for him to say, "Hi!" We continued in a similar way on a week-to-week basis, role-playing all new responses in a variety of ways, reversing roles so that he could observe the response done "properly," and discussing any possible difficulties in detail. For example, it took an entire fifty-minute session for him to learn how to make a two-minute call to ask a woman for a date. The rapid improvement which took

---

[1] Most behavior modifiers would attribute the success of this approach primarily to various conditioning factors which affect the patient's behavior. Among these are *positive reinforcement* (the desirable environmental consequences following each new step), *shaping* (reaching a complex response by successively closer approximations), and *generalization* (making the newly acquired response in a variety of situations other than the setting in which it was learned).

49

place in his contacts with women is probably attributable mainly to the little-by-little approach. At the same time, however, his ability to master the weekly tasks despite his anxiety and initial pessimism as well as the rapidity of his progress suggest that the placebo value of the ritual was also important. In other words, his improvement is comparable to that of a person who takes an effective pill for his illness but gets well "too fast" because of his faith in the pill.

Another important healing ritual, which is associated primarily with communications therapy, involves the surprising strategy of telling a patient to continue doing what he is doing (practice his problem) so as to get him to stop doing it. Although there are a number of ingenious explanations for the success of this ritual (among them, double bind communications theory, the social psychological theory of reactance, and the behavioral concepts of extinction and reactive inhibition—all described in references listed in the Annotated Bibliography), it can most easily be seen as analogous to the maneuver of parents who get their negativistic child to bed by telling him that he must stay up. In addition, the instruction to "do what you're doing" is helpful in overcoming patients' feelings of being out of control. In other words, when they practice their problem deliberately, they are acting voluntarily rather than in an uncontrolled way.

This healing ritual can be illustrated by the treatment of a man who squandered his paycheck each Friday by buying drinks for everyone at a series of bars and getting drunk himself. The therapist had the man list the bars he went to in sequence, the number of rounds of drinks he ordered for others at each bar, and the number of drinks (and what kind) he had at each bar. The therapist then instructed the man to follow the list exactly after receiving his next paycheck. At the next session, the man stated that he had gone home sober before completing the list. Apparently, the therapist's instructions had taken all the fun out of his spree.

In this ritual, the placebo approach helps to persuade patients to agree to practice their problems. If asked to do so without any special explanation, patients typically consider the therapist to be the crazy one and refuse to follow the suggestion on the grounds that they are trying to cure, not exacerbate, their problems. Thus, the therapist must devise a rationale in order to get patients to go along with his instructions. For example, in the above illustration, the therapist might explain to the patient that as part of the diagnostic phase of therapy he needs to know exactly what the patient feels from moment to moment while on his bender and therefore would like the patient to write down his feelings just before ordering each drink. In this way, the patient's belief in the importance of helping his therapist to make an accurate diagnosis enables him to follow a useful but peculiar ritual.

The following description of a part of the treatment of a difficult case illustrates a number of points discussed in this chapter. The patient was a rather gloomy young man in his sophomore year at college who had already switched his major field of study several times. He spoke of his problems in a boring monotone and explained minor or irrelevant points in great detail. Some of the problems that he wanted help with were his poor work in school, his lack of interest in academia, and his general feelings of depression and purposelessness. (Though we also worked on other difficulties, they are not relevant to the present illustration.) As I spoke with him, I realized that he had left many responsibilities unmet in both his academic and his personal life. I concluded that his excessive worrying about details had created a situation in which he could not decide what to do first. Furthermore, I hypothesized that his inability to accomplish even minor tasks had diminished his already low self-esteem, made him feel that he could never successfully complete his schoolwork, and led to his hopeless feelings. I based my healing ritual on this formulation, and after a persuasive explanation of the therapeutic value of my approach, I worked with him to list on index cards every task which he needed to accomplish, from washing his laundry to writing his term papers. I then had him arrange the cards in the order of difficulty of the tasks for him. Finally, I gave him the three easiest cards and asked him to complete the tasks before our next weekly session. The following week, after I had praised him for his accomplishments, we discarded the cards listing completed tasks and made up new ones for tasks that had come up during the preceding week. Once these had been placed in their proper order, I assigned him the four easiest tasks to complete.

The goals of this little-by-little ritual were to enable him to get a feeling of accomplishment and to diminish the number of things he worried about. I hoped that, as we approached the difficult school-related items, he would have the confidence to tackle them. If he did so, I thought that he might well discover some aspect of his schoolwork which he enjoyed and give me a lead to how school might become more meaningful (and life less purposeless) for him. With this idea in mind, I also had him take a vocational interest test.

At first, the results of therapy seemed encouraging because he was able to complete the assigned tasks. However, the successes ended abruptly when we reached the school-related items. The patient's weak excuses for not even attempting some of the simple tasks (such as choosing a topic for a term paper) made me suspect that my assessment —and hence the therapeutic ritual—might be incorrect. I therefore began the assessment process anew, in an attempt to discover the reason for the sudden end to his improvement.

As we talked about the patient's schoolwork, he told

me that his parents were quite worried about his performance. He said that they were afraid that he would flunk out, be drafted, and then die in Viet Nam. As he mentioned his parents' fears, I noticed that he smiled faintly. When I asked him about his facial expression, he denied that he had smiled. In doing so, however, he smiled again. I pointed this out to him and asked whether it was possible that he enjoyed the way in which his poor work was upsetting his parents. Though he had, by then, become aware that he was smiling, he insisted that the smile had no significance. In addition, he became quite emphatic about how much he wanted to do well in school and how sorry he was that his parents were upset. The more he denied that he enjoyed upsetting his parents, though, the more he smiled. In fact, he occasionally burst into embarrassed laughter.

This unexpected display of merriment led me to hypothesize that since the patient was a rather dutiful son, he had learned to use personal failure as a way of retaliating for the unpleasant experience of conforming to his parents' demands. In other words, his smile appeared to reflect his satisfaction at having successfully failed.

Because a paper was due for one of his courses before the following session, I decided to try a new approach to his problem based on my new assessment. Using a variation of the do-what-you're-doing strategy, I told him to write the paper and tell his parents that he had not. True to the new formulation, he smiled when I made the suggestion. Although he said—laughingly—that he could not possibly hurt his parents that way, I insisted on the importance of his following my instructions and explained how much we could learn from what happened.

When he returned the following week, he told me that he had written the paper. This success contrasted dramatically with his previous inability even to decide upon a topic and lent further credence to the new assessment. However, I soon discovered that he had decided to spend the weekend with his parents. Because his parents' apartment was rather small, he had been forced to write the paper in their presence. Thus, he had been unable to tell them that he did not do it. In other words, he responded to my instructions with the same technique that he used on his parents: In the process of writing the paper, he simultaneously let me down. Naturally, the way in which the second ritual succeeded introduced new complications into his treatment, but they are not relevant here.

In summary, this case fragment illustrates a number of important applications of placebo principles to directive psychotherapy. Among these are the way in which the healing ritual grows out of the therapist's formulation of the patient's problems and beliefs, the consequent need for an accurate assessment of those problems and beliefs, the failure of a healing ritual as a signal to the therapist that his assessment was incorrect, a new assessment leading to a new ritual, and the "correct" ritual leading to a rapid improvement in the problem it is aimed at. In addition, the presentation provided further illustrations of both the little-by-little and the do-what-you're-doing healing rituals.

FIVE

~~~~~~~~~~~~~~~~~~~~~~~~~~~~~

Maintaining the Cure

~~~~~~~~~~~~~~~~~~~~~~~~~~~~~

Because of its emphasis on self-cure, the process of placebo therapy increasingly stresses the patient's interactions with the environment while simultaneously diminishing the importance of his interactions with the therapist. In emphasizing assessment and the therapeutic contract, the pretherapy stage is concerned almost exclusively with interactions between patient and therapist. Although the therapy stage involves the therapist's telling the patient what to do and checking on what he has done, the patient takes the equally important responsibility of using the healing ritual to cure himself. Therefore, when the time for terminating therapy arrives, the groundwork has already been laid for the patient to make a smooth transition back into a life without therapy. This kind of therapy contrasts dramatically with the sort of long-term therapy that encourages regression. Given the dependence on the therapist which is fostered during the year-in-year-out life with therapy, it is not surprising that termination is frequently a difficult emotional experience for patients; and they often continue to doubt their ability to function on their own long after therapy has ended.

As has been emphasized in discussing the other stages of psychotherapy, the therapist should structure termination so as to make it a therapeutic event. The importance of his last contact with his patient is illustrated by the fact that, although much of therapy becomes a blur in a former patient's memory, he often recalls vividly some aspect of his last session. One therapist who was analyzed by Jung told me on three different occasions the master's parting words of advice to him but mentioned few other momentous events in his analysis. Because a therapist wants to ensure that his patient will not be uncured by the environment as rapidly as he was cured by therapy, the following discussion is aimed at elucidating some of the ways in which the therapist can use his final contact with the patient to further his goal.

A person entering therapy is often entangled in a vicious circle of self-aggravating problems. For example, his low self-esteem may make him feel incapable of accomplishing anything, and this feeling may in turn lead him to try less hard to meet life's daily challenges. His diminished efforts naturally lead to failures, and his experience of failure tends to decrease further his already low self-esteem. Placebo therapy attempts to break this circle. The new behavior and beliefs which arise from the healing ritual lead to an upsurge of hope, which in turn promotes the sequence of zeal, success, and increased self-esteem. The strategy of the therapy stage, which aims at creating a self-perpetuating virtuous circle, involves the following: helping the patient to develop new behavior and beliefs, strengthening the new behavior and beliefs, strengthening the patient's ability to cope with challenges to his new behavior and beliefs, and getting the patient to act in a manner ensuring that others will respond positively to his new behavior and beliefs.

Once the virtuous circle has been securely set into motion, the therapist should step out of its way and terminate therapy. His parting placebo communication—"Congratulations! You've cured yourself."—contains a number of therapeutic farewell messages. The most important of these are "you're cured (you're not crazy)"; "you've done it yourself (you're not out of control because you've mastered your own problems)"; and "I'm pleased with and impressed by what you've accomplished, and you should to be too."

A number of elements in placebo therapy serve to maintain the virtuous circle after therapy has ended. Figure 2, a schematic postview of placebo therapy, focuses on these elements. It emphasizes the interactions of the patient's new beliefs and new behavior with each other and with the environment in a complex and self-perpetuating manner. Although such a diagram obviously cannot include all the rel-

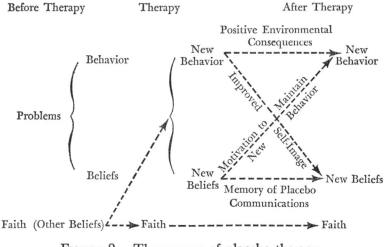

FIGURE 2. The process of placebo therapy.

evant interactions, it should clarify the kinds of forces which maintain the cure after termination.

If the therapist has been ingenious enough to get the patient to develop new behavior which leads to positive consequences, the new behavior will persist. This well-established operant principle enables the successful therapist to end therapy with confidence. In addition to these environmental forces, however, the patient's feelings of self-mastery, his new self-confidence, his more optimistic world view (that is, his feeling that the world is a place where he can influence his own destiny), and his other new beliefs both strengthen his new behavior during good times and maintain it during transient periods of environmental adversity. Similarly, the patient's self-enhancing awareness that he is able to behave in a fulfilling manner and that his new behavior is well received by the environment act reciprocally to strengthen his new beliefs. Furthermore, his emotionally charged memory of the potent words of his therapist's placebo communications serves to maintain his new beliefs when he encounters situations which tend to contradict them. One commonly hears former traditional therapy patients criticize themselves with such statements as "my therapist told me it is self-destructive for me to do this"; former placebo therapy patients are more likely to reward themselves with "my therapist was right when he said that I have the strength to achieve this."

At the same time that Figure 2 indicates what is changed by placebo therapy, it points up what is not changed. The patient's faith—his strong beliefs which are not part of his problem—remains the same, for leaving the patient's faith untouched (or even strengthening it) is a key placebo principle. Its importance is evident in the therapist's attempt to demonstrate to his patient an inconsistency between his problem beliefs and his faith, thereby compelling him to alter his beliefs. Once his beliefs have changed, however, and after therapy has ended, the consistency of the patient's faith with his new beliefs serves as an additional support for these beliefs.

The issue of termination highlights certain distinctive features of the placebo approach. In traditional psychotherapy, the therapist assumes that the patient's difficulties arise from an imbalance among intrapsychic forces. Once those forces are realigned (however long the realignment may take), the patient is ready to leave therapy; and it is assumed that his new psychic strength will enable him to function on his own. In placebo therapy, no such assumption is made. The posttherapy environment plays an important role in the therapist's planning, and he makes extensive preparations for the patient's return to a life without therapy. This difference in style of termination—direct and short-term versus indirect and long-term—is characteristic of other differences between placebo therapy and traditional therapy. In the former, the therapist makes assessments directly rather than waiting for material to emerge; he institutes a healing ritual rather than waiting for the patient to grow; he monitors the patient's progress rather than waiting for him to learn haphazardly; and he terminates once the goals have been reached rather than waiting for the patient to outgrow his need for therapy. It is this planned directness which distinguishes the placebo approach from traditional therapy and makes it possible to deal in a brief period with crucial issues which are often overlooked in the course of longer but less structured treatment.

The techniques of termination are essentially adaptations of other placebo principles. The two most important techniques are congratulating the patient on his self-cure and making final preparations for the patient's return to a life without therapy. Throughout treatment, the therapist shows interest in, agrees with, approves of, and otherwise rewards the patient's statements that he has improved. Naturally, at termination, it is especially important for the therapist to elicit and reward such statements so that the patient can demonstrate to himself, with his therapist's approval, that he really is cured. Once he believes that he is cured, it is a simple matter for him to leave therapy.

Therapists sometimes object to this optimistic approach to the patient's statements on the grounds that it leads patients to become unrealistic in their self-evaluations. This objection is based on a failure to distinguish between a patient's observing his behavior accurately and labeling that behavior. It is always desirable for a person to observe accurately both his own behavior and the responses of others to what he says and does. The entire placebo approach involves strengthening the patient's ability to make such observations, and this ability is one of the main factors which maintain the cure after termination. Thus, if a patient knows what he does that leads people to treat him in an unpleasant manner, he can choose whether his present behavior or the reactions of others are more important to him in a given situation. Observing one's own behavior is, however, both logically and descriptively distinct from labeling it. Whether one considers a particular act to be good, bad, neurotic, psychotic, creative, hopeful, self-actualizing, regressive, dependent, naive, masochistic, loving, warm, cold, expressive, rigid, bungling, exploitative, or ambivalent is quite distinct from what that act is. However, an evaluative label has consequences for the individual fully as significant as the consequences of the behavior itself. Therefore, throughout treatment, the therapist strives to make the patient label himself and his behavior in a positive (or at least hopeful) manner while simultaneously observing his behavior accurately. This dual approach is illustrated in the following interaction: Therapist: "How have things been going this past week?" Patient: "Much better." Therapist: "I'm glad to hear that." Patient: "My boss has been giving me hell, though." Therapist: "What happened?"

In this conversation, the therapist rewarded the patient's labeling of himself as improved. When the patient then said something to indicate that he might in fact be worse, the therapist did not respond, "There you go with your rose-colored glasses again! How can things be much better when your boss has been giving you hell?" Instead, he began an exploration of what the boss did, what the patient did, and what the patient might have done differently. In other words, the therapist encouraged the patient both to label his behavior positively and to observe it accurately so that he could learn from it for the future. When a therapist acts in this manner, he transmits the placebo communication "even though things are good now, it's possible for you to make them still better."

The only change in the therapist's technique as termination nears is a shift from encouraging statements of improvement to encouraging statements of cure. One of the most effective ways to make the shift is for the therapist to refer to the therapeutic contract and point out that the goals have been met. Once the patient agrees that they have in fact been met, the therapist can ask the patient the key question, "Is there anything else you'd like to work on?" If either the patient or the therapist can think of a new, mutually acceptable goal, a further contract can be developed. If neither one can, the end of therapy is at hand. I have often seen, at this point, an expression of insight appear on the patient's face. Because he has already agreed that he has nothing further to work on, the awareness of that fact cannot be responsible for the new expression. My impression is that the patient has made the connection "if I don't need therapy, then it must be that I'm no longer neurotic!" Naturally, if he expressed his feelings of mental health at this point, I would agree with him.

Although the entire process of placebo therapy involves preparing the patient for a life without therapy, a number of specific messages enhancing the preparations can be communicated to the patient during the last session.

61

Some of these, which have already been discussed, include: attributing the patient's future difficulties to "life's ups and downs" rather than to "mental illness"; reminding the patient that he can always return to see the therapist if he is troubled by new problems while reassuring him that he is unlikely to need further therapy; and pointing out to the patient that, if and when he does have further problems, he can think up self-mastery techniques on his own. (If the patient does return, the therapist can take the role of consultant in developing a self-mastery technique and sidestep involvement with the "mental illness" label. Furthermore, the unsuccessful self-mastery techniques initiated by the patient and the ways in which they failed provide useful information for a new assessment.)

An additional technique involves preparing the patient with ways to interpret his new behavior to others. Typically, when a person starts acting in a noticeably different manner, his friends and associates are uncertain about how to respond to him. Because it is important for them to respond positively to his new behavior, the patient must work to encourage that response. And, just as the therapist's explanations helped the patient to change his behavior, his own explanations can help to change the behavior of others toward him. In particular, the patient must persuade others to accept his new behavior and view it as characteristic of him.

If the patient is to do so, he must use a little placebo therapy of his own by basing his explanations on an understanding of others' beliefs about how people change. For example, many people make a distinction between "real change" and "superficial change," so the patient must convince such people that his change is real. I once chatted with a colleague who felt he was getting nowhere in his interactions with a few other therapists. He wished to try relating to them in a completely different manner but felt that they would be suspicious of an abrupt change on his part. Both he and the other therapists were psychoanalytically oriented, so I suggested that he spread the word of some "meaningful developments" in his personal analysis at about the time he changed his behavior toward them. Because the therapists were analytically oriented, it was possible for them to label change resulting from psychoanalysis as "real." Their acceptance of my colleague's new behavior also enabled it to succeed (and be "real") where it might otherwise have failed (and been "superficial").

In a similar manner, if a patient's friends believe in therapy, he can attribute his new behavior to the therapeutic process. If, however, his friends believe that therapy is ineffective and that anyone who enters therapy is crazy, it would be foolhardy for him to mention that he had consulted a therapist. Instead, he might attribute his new behavior to the salutary effects of a vacation, a raise, the discovery of new meaning in his marriage, or an uplifting sermon in church. The choice of explanation for his new behavior could even vary from person to person as long as the explainees were unlikely to get together. For example, the patient might develop one standard explanation for colleagues at work and another for acquaintances or relatives.

Because a therapist using placebo principles commonly asks how others are responding to or might respond to a given behavior, there is nothing unusual about making such an inquiry toward the end of therapy. If the patient's answer suggests that he may have difficulty in getting others to accept his new behavior, the therapist should discuss the situation with him. On occasion it may even be desirable to role play the explanation with him; a hesitant explanation by the patient encourages the sort of doubts in others which he wishes to prevent, and role-playing can give him a chance to practice speaking in a convincing manner.

Although no case study can illustrate all the placebo principles, the following case does give a general feeling for the beginning-to-end process of therapy. The case is particularly interesting not only because treatment consisted almost exclusively of placebo communications but also because of the evident negative effect of other communications on the patient's problems.

I first saw Portnoy A. in a university psychological center during fall registration. He was a tall, thin, worried-looking sophomore who spoke in an excessively sincere voice —in short, a *very* good boy. He began the discussion of his need for therapy by asking me to write a note to the Registrar stating that he was neurotic and requesting that he be permitted to enroll in less than a full-time program because of his psychological impairment. As we spoke further, the history of his difficulties began to emerge.

During the previous spring term, Portnoy had been quite unhappy. His roommates in the dormitory had been antagonistic toward him—which was not surprising, considering that he was such a square—and he had had few friends and no girl friends. He felt lonely and insecure, and these feelings in turn made it difficult for him to concentrate on his studies. As a result, his academic work suffered, and his diminished school performance made him doubt himself still more. Eventually, he sought help at the psychological center and was seen by a therapist for six sessions during the second half of the spring term. The therapist's notes indicated that, in addition to the above problems, Portnoy was worried that he might be a latent homosexual—although this topic never came up in our meetings.

After the term ended, he returned to New York City for the summer to the infantilizing overprotection of smother love. Despite his upbringing, a year in college had led him to become somewhat self-reliant, and his minor expressions of independence at home horrified his parents. When he told his mother that he had been unhappy at college, she put two and two together and recognized that only a specialist could help her poor baby. (Such mothers are frequently expert at

finding the *right* specialist; and even if the specialist says
something that she does not want to hear, she can misunder-
stand him or consult a "more competent" specialist.)

Mrs. A's first step was to take her son to a neurologist,
who prescribed some pills. In speaking of the visit, Portnoy
reported impressively, "That doctor said I was neurotic, and
he had an office on Park Avenue!"

Next, his mother took him to a well-known social
agency, where a psychologist gave him some tests. Portnoy
later returned to discuss the test results; and he told me that
the following interaction took place during that discussion:
Psychologist: "Would you say that you're normal or neurotic?" Portnoy: "Normal." Psychologist: "Wrong! Neurotic." The psychologist went on to tell him that he was too
neurotic to return to college and that he should live with his
parents, begin long-term psychotherapy, and take a few
courses at night school.

Although his mother had been able to marshal an
impressive array of evidence that it was he (and not she)
who was crazy, Portnoy recognized that he was at least as
miserable at home as he had been at school. Therefore, despite his having been shaken by his contacts with specialists,
he decided to resume his studies. He proposed to his mother
that he return to the university, take only a small number of
easy courses, and continue in therapy at the university psychological center. I do not know why his mother accepted
this solution, but some of the following arguments likely
played a part in her thinking: (1) Because the specialist
ploy had enabled her to win her main battle with her son,
she could afford the largesse of acceding to his request. (2)
Whether her son's behavior was attributed to adolescence,
independence, or neurosis, he was still no pleasure to live
with; and with him away at college, she could have some
peace. (3) Therapy at the university is free. (4) If his return
to college did not work out, he could always come home and
follow the psychologist's advice.

As the background to Portnoy's problems emerged, it became evident that he was genuinely worried that he would be unable to handle a full schedule of courses. He had registered for the minimum number of credits necessary to remain a full-time student and had been told that he would need a professional's note to be permitted to take fewer courses.

When I inquired into Portnoy's present circumstances, however, the picture became much brighter. He had only one roommate instead of two, and the roommate seemed congenial. Of course, Portnoy pointed out anxiously, it was quite possible that dormitory troubles might develop as the term progressed. In a similar manner, he indicated that his academic program seemed easy to handle, but he was worried that his neurosis might get the better of him by mid-term. He also indicated that he had joined a club where he could share his interests with other students. Although he had hopes of making friends there, he remembered the loneliness of the previous term and was afraid that, as people got to know him more, they would like him less.

In planning treatment from the above information, the following considerations were uppermost in my mind: The environmental conditions which had made Portnoy miserable seemed to be largely absent; his desire to make friends, do well in school, and avoid returning home constituted excellent motivation for change; and his insecurity and tendency to worry even when things were going well seemed to be the most appropriate target for treatment. The third point was a reason for real concern because his acting on his insecurity and worry could recreate the problems of the previous term. If he used his neurosis as a reason for demanding special considerations from his roommate, Portnoy could antagonize him and wind up with another hostile roommate. Similarly, his worrying that he might do poorly in school could interfere with his studying and begin a vicious circle of academic deterioration.

The danger that such problems would materialize is particularly evident if Portnoy's case is viewed from the standpoint of one of the forms of therapy relying primarily on "insight." One possible disastrous course for such therapy might be as follows: As Portnoy explores his feelings of loneliness, he begins to examine his desire for a girl friend. He attributes his failure with women to his feelings of inadequacy and considers the possibility that he may be a latent homosexual. He then begins to explore his relationship with his mother and its effect on his view of women. Until now he had thought of himself as a dutiful son who loved his mother. However, as he talks further, he is surprised to find himself expressing considerable resentment and anger toward her. Eventually, he realizes that he hates his mother for keeping him dependent on her and therefore must want to avoid such a castastrophe with other women. This analysis leads him to the self-destructive "insight" that he really is a latent homosexual. Although such a thought is unpleasant, it relieves him of the responsibility for initiating further anxiety-ridden contacts with women. At this point therapy becomes twice as difficult because the therapist must deal with this new and powerful belief, and the possibility of Portnoy's considering actual homosexual experimentation becomes a real one. In a similar manner, such therapy might arouse the worry that he has a need to fail or the feeling that he wants to do well just to please his mother—either of which would undoubtedly impair his school performance. Because Portnoy was something of a psychic hypochondriac and because he was earnest enough to see any therapy through to the bitter end, I felt that the danger of his getting caught in a pointless and interminable self-exploration was a real one. (As psychoanalytically oriented therapists can see, Portnoy met all the criteria for a good candidate for analysis of an obsessional neurosis.) I therefore proceeded instead to encourage his moves toward independence and to modify his style of worrying and his belief that he was neurotic.

I reasoned that, because specialists had been able to shake Portnoy's view of himself, his faith in specialists must be a potent one. I therefore assumed the stance of a confident professional and told Portnoy that he did not seem particularly neurotic to me. He invoked Park Avenue again, and his glance around the counseling center office expressed a rather disdainful comparison with the sumptuous locations of his previous diagnoses. Nevertheless, I remained unimpressed with his mental illness. I explained that it appeared that he had been unhappy at school the previous term because of his roommates and unhappy at home because of his mother. Now that he no longer had to live in upsetting circumstances, it was natural that he was not upset. The reason that the two professionals had mistakenly thought he was neurotic was that they had seen him while he was in an upset state. I went on to say that, because he was neither neurotic nor upset now and because I agreed with his own feeling that he could handle his course work, there was no reason for me to write a note requesting permission for him to take less than a full-time program. If difficulties arose in the future, I could always discuss the possibility of writing a note for him at that time.

Even though my communications contradicted those of other specialists, Portnoy was receptive to mine for several reasons. First, the other professionals had merely labeled his behavior "neurotic," while I not only labeled it "not neurotic" but also explained my reasoning as well as the others' "mistaken" reasoning. Then, by taking his side against his mother, I became more trustworthy. Finally, because my message was a reassuring one, it was relatively easy to accept. Nevertheless, his promise to his mother to enter therapy as well as his style of worrying meant that there was more for me to do than to state my message once. I therefore indicated that, although he did not appear neurotic to me, I would be willing to continue to meet with him once a week to see whether there was anything we could find that was worth working on in therapy.

Under my sincere and interested guidance, we spent the next three sessions assiduously looking for problems. Each time we thought we had one, it turned out not to be a problem—and I used the nonproblem to show Portnoy that he was worried over nothing. He worried that he would not be able to function away from home, but as the weeks passed he found that he was doing fine. He worried that he and his roommate would not continue to get on, but no catastrophe occurred. He worried that he would be unable to decide on a subject to major in, but he enjoyed the economics courses he was taking and decided to major in that field. Finally, he worried about having no friends; but just as we were about to settle on finding friends as a goal, he made a few friends in the club he had joined.

In addition to showing that his stated worries were not really problems, I attempted to deal with his unstated worry. Thus, while we were discussing the problem of loneliness, I casually remarked that men sometimes misinterpret their natural need for male friends as latent homosexuality. I said that putting an arm around a buddy's shoulders while drinking beer or slapping a teammate on the behind during a football game is a form of masculine comradeship—and it is a shame that some men deny themselves this kind of friendship because of their anxiety about latent homosexuality. Because this comment was made in the abstract and could not refer to him (he had never mentioned homosexuality), he did not even respond to it. However, his reporting in the fourth session that he had a girl friend suggested that my words might well have reassured him about his masculinity.

By the end of the fourth session, Portnoy and I had given up on finding a problem worth therapeutic attention. When I assured him that if such a problem were to arise I would be glad to work on it in therapy, he agreed to terminate.

Over the next five months, on two or three occasions I received a message at the psychological center that Portnoy wished to speak to me. Each time I called him back he was not in; and before I could try again the next day, I received a message that he did not need to see me after all. Finally, during the spring term I received one more such message, and this time he answered the phone when I returned his call. Following through on my promise to be available if he needed me, I set up a time for an interview.

Portnoy began the session by stating that all the problems for which he had consulted me the previous term, including loneliness and difficulty with his studies, were gone. However, he said that he had two new problems he wanted to discuss. The first was that during vacation he occasionally got tension around his eyes that prevented him from reading. The tension occurred while he was at home with his nagging parents but disappeared after he returned to school. However, he was worried that he might get the tension again and that it might prevent him from studying. I told him that, if the tension returned, I would be glad to teach him relaxation exercises for his eyes to make it go away. He seemed satisfied with this offer and appeared confident that the exercises would take care of the tension. His second problem was that he occasionally got so excited about the club activities that he got a mild stomach ache. He not only said that it was harder to study when he had a stomach ache but also was worried that his stomach aches might become more severe. The following conversation then took place: Me: "Have you tried Tums?" Portnoy: "You don't understand! This is a psychosomatic symptom!" Me: "I know. And Tums are quite effective." Portnoy: (Silence.) Me: "Of course, you could always try bicarbonate of soda." Portnoy: "I'd rather use Tums because you can carry them in your pocket. . . . But you don't seem to think I have a problem." Me: "You do have a problem. You worry too much. Stop worrying!"

We spent the rest of the session discussing the minor

problems which arise as a part of life (life's ups and downs) and concluded that, though they are inevitable, they are not severe and are no cause for worry. Our previous sessions had already made Portnoy aware of his tendency to worry, so he could see what I was talking about. He also admitted that the unpleasantness at home during vacation had led his mother to insist that he needed someone to talk to (that is, a therapist to beat him into submission). I told him that, although she might think he needed someone to talk to, I did not think so and that it was pointless for him to enter therapy just to pacify her.

Portnoy seemed to have gotten my message, but I thought he might return in the future with one or two new worries, until he became used to functioning on his own. However, he did not request another session. I ran into him about a year later while I was walking across the campus and (for what it is worth), when I said, "How goes it?" he answered with a smile, "Fine."

This case is real therapy, placebo therapy. Although the chain of events may seem quite simple, the results were dramatic. In five sessions a young man who had been doing poorly in college began doing well and chose a major field of study; his loneliness was replaced with a girl friend and a number of male friends; and his self-doubt, worry, and fears that he was neurotic were markedly diminished. Even though there was still room for improvement in his relationship with his parents, he had, by the end of therapy, come to see his moves toward independence in a positive light. Thus, at the time of termination I felt that it was better to keep him out of therapy, where he could cope with his parental difficulties when they occurred, than to emphasize the importance of his parents or reward his dependency with the unending support of long-term psychotherapy.

Even though a therapeutic contract was never actually arranged, moves toward making such a contract served two important purposes in Portnoy's treatment. First, the repeated failure to find a problem needing therapeutic attention was an effective method of conveying to Portnoy that he was not crazy, did not need therapy, and was merely getting himself worked up over minor difficulties. The other area in which the contract was involved was Portnoy's initial request for a letter to the Registrar. If I had written such a letter, I would have undermined his chance to learn that he was capable of functioning successfully in school; even if he did well in a curtailed program, Portnoy could still retain his belief that he would have failed (both psychologically and academically) with a full-time schedule. I would also have strengthened his dependency by demonstrating that therapists, like parents, come to his rescue whenever the going gets rough and diminished his incentive to master difficulties on his own. Finally, it is generally a poor idea for a therapist to agree to a patient's offer of "I'll see you in therapy if you'll do X for me." This offer can be tempting, particularly when it involves money (for example, "I'll enter long-term psychotherapy if you'll write a letter to my draft board to get me out of the army"), but such a contract leads to a travesty of therapy in which progress is all but impossible. The reason is that, once the patient improves, he must be drafted or take more courses or otherwise suffer; that is, the continuation of "therapy" is contingent upon the patient's making no progress.

Although it would have been a mistake for me to write the letter for Portnoy, it would also have been wrong to refuse to write it because of the danger of the following type of interaction: Patient: "I'll see you in therapy if you'll do X for me." Therapist: "I won't do X for you." Patient: "Then I won't see you in therapy." Instead of accepting or denying such a request, a therapist does best to treat it as an initial ploy in the process of arriving at a contract. Because my strategy with Portnoy involved demonstrating to him that he did not need therapy, it was both easy and appropriate for me to defer his request to a later date. In schematic form, the interaction is as follows: Patient: "I'll see you in therapy if you'll do X for me." Therapist: "First let's discuss whether or not you need therapy and whether or not you need X."

My last observation concerning Portnoy's treatment is that the main placebo communication consisted of my telling him that he was not neurotic. The effectiveness of this communication resulted largely from his faith in the words of specialists. And, though I did everything I could to change his belief that he was neurotic, I was equally careful not to challenge his faith in specialists. In other words, this case provides a clear illustration of the way in which placebo therapy uses one set of a patient's beliefs (his faith) to change another set of his beliefs (his problems).

The next four chapters deal with the therapeutic application of placebo principles in different types of psychotherapy. In particular, the effectiveness of hypnotherapy, behavior modification, and group therapy appears to be easily enhanceable by the use of placebo principles. Furthermore, persuasive communcations directed to mass audiences affect both their members' self-images and their attitudes toward mental health; and the last of these chapters suggests ways to make such effects more salutary.

SIX

Applications to Hypnotherapy

Placebo principles can be applied to any form of psychotherapy that is consistent with them and thereby enhance the effect, if any, of the therapy alone. Hypnotherapy provides an ideal setting for the application of such principles because hypnosis is a potent form of socially sanctioned magic in our culture and readily inspires the sort of faith which can be mobilized for healing purposes.

Because this book is a manual of psychotherapy, not of hypnosis, an extensive review of hypnotic principles and techniques would be inappropriate here.[1] However, the fol-

[1] Suggested readings in hypnosis are included in the Annotated Bibliography.

lowing brief discussion of hypnosis should provide the familiarity necessary to understand the ways in which placebo principles can be applied to hypnotherapy.

Hypnosis is an unusual situation in which a subject is asked by a hypnotist to do strange things or experience strange events. Most people are surprised to find that they can do or experience many of the phenomena which are suggested to them; and they tend to attribute their unusual performance to the powers of the hypnotist or the magic of the trance state. It is easy to understand such attributions; the hypnotic experience is an unusual one, and ready explanations for one's performance have already been provided by society. However, the most important causes of people's responsiveness to hypnotic suggestions are quite different.

Researchers have found that a surprising number of people respond to "hypnotic" suggestions without the benefit of the hocus-pocus associated with hypnosis. In other words, much of what is called "hypnotic" looks difficult to do—because it is unusual—but actually is easy for many people. For example, consider the following suggestion: "Let's see how good your imagination is. Most people, if they imagine their right arm to be as light as a helium balloon, find that it will float right up into the air. Why don't you try it?" Many subjects will be pleasantly surprised to find their right arms floating.

The responsiveness to suggestions can, however, be increased or decreased in a number of ways. One is the wording of the suggestion. For example, if the arm levitation suggestion had begun with the words "let's see how gullible you are," relatively few people would have responded. In addition, some suggestions are harder to respond to than others. Many fewer people would respond to a suggestion to see George Washington alive before them than to the arm levitation suggestion. It should be emphasized, however, that a positive response to even so difficult a suggestion is neither especially rare nor "sick."

Saying that some suggestions are more difficult than others is really another way of saying that some people are more suggestible than others. Thus, people who are able to respond to a difficult suggestion are more suggestible than those who cannot. In fact, tests of hypnotizability consist of a series of increasingly difficult suggestions; and a person's hypnotizability score is simply the number of suggestions to which he is able to respond.

One of the ways in which a hypnotist can increase a subject's responsiveness to test suggestions is to precede them with a hypnotic induction. The hypnotist may, for example, tell the subject to stare at a fixed spot on a wall and then suggest that his eyelids are closing and that he is becoming relaxed and drowsy. Although a hypnotic induction may help a subject enter a trance state, other explanations for his increased responsiveness to suggestions are conceivable.

An alternative explanation can be deduced from the fact that inductions typically involve easy-to-follow suggestions. For example, when a person stares at a spot, his eyes naturally get tired; and it is quite easy to relax in response to a suggestion of relaxation. When the subject sees that he is responding to the hypnotic induction, he "realizes" that he must be hypnotized—and must therefore be able to follow the hypnotist's other suggestions. Similarly, motivating instructions (that is, telling the subject that he will find it easy to respond and encouraging him to try hard) are just as effective as a hypnotic induction in increasing responsiveness.

The argument over whether a trance state exists continues to preoccupy researchers. However, as far as hypnotherapy is concerned, it makes no difference whether or not the trance state exists; therapists are primarily concerned with knowing how to make patients change their behavior, not with why what they do works. Thus, all researchers in hypnosis (whether or not they believe in the existence of a trance state) agree with the above principles governing responsiveness to suggestions. Their only disagreement is over whether or not the concept of a trance state is necessary to explain why responsiveness varies in these lawful ways. Thus, the above principles constitute a body of knowledge which can be used in amplifying the effectiveness of placebo communications, and the framework of placebo therapy can be applied to those principles in constructing potent hypnotic healing rituals. The remainder of this chapter is devoted to elaborating on these interactions between hypnosis and placebo therapy.

In a very real and important sense, every interpersonal communication includes an element of suggestion. Such suggestions (that is, "do X") may be as simple as "believe what I'm telling you" but are typically more complicated. The nature of a given suggestion depends upon the people involved, the situation, the words of the communication, and the nonverbal qualifications of those words.[2] For example, consider a man at the wheel of the family car whose wife, sitting next to him, says, "The light is green." Depending on the context of the remark and its nonverbal qualifications, her suggestion may be "look at the light," "start driving," "stop daydreaming," "listen to me," or even "stop talking about what you were saying before I interrupted to tell you that the light is green." Whether or not her husband responds to her suggestion is determined by a number of variables, including such "hypnotic" factors as the difficulty of the suggestion and the level of his hypnotizability. In other words, elements of suggestion and respon-

---

[2] A more detailed discussion of the subject from another point of view can be found in the works by Jay Haley and other communications therapists. Appropriate references appear in the Annotated Bibliography.

siveness are at work wherever people are together; and, if a therapist can harness these omnipresent forces, he can use them to achieve therapeutic goals.

Once a therapist realizes that everything he says to his patients includes suggestions,[3] he can increase his effectiveness by keeping the following questions in mind: What do I want to suggest? How can I form my suggestion so that my patient will be most likely to respond? The answer to the first question can be inferred from the goals of the therapeutic contract. The therapist can use his words to suggest either general improvement or a particular step in the direction of one of the goals. In answering the second question, all the principles of placebo therapy are relevant. In addition, however, knowledge about hypnosis can be applied to maximize the impact of the therapist's communications. For example, both the use of motivating instructions and the careful wording of suggestions would increase the likelihood of a patient's responding positively.

Besides making deliberate use of direct suggestions throughout the course of therapy, the therapist can devise specific hypnotic healing rituals for particular problems. Because self-hypnosis is consonant with the aim of self-cure, it is an ideal vehicle for such rituals.

The first step in devising a hypnotic healing ritual is to find out how hypnotizable the patient is, which can easily be done with any standardized hypnotic induction. Once a therapist knows how responsive his patient is, he can vary his technique accordingly. Also, by communicating "I want to find out how hypnotizable you are" instead of "I'm going to hypnotize you," the therapist sets up a situation in which he cannot fail. Thus, if the patient responds to none of his suggestions, the therapist can say, "Fine. It appears that you

[3] Naturally, everything a patient says contains suggestions too. When a therapist asserts that he has learned a lot from his patients, he means that his patients have changed him. This change is inevitable and—depending on how the therapist has changed—usually desirable.

are not hypnotizable, which means that we will do X." In other words, the therapist has succeeded in assessing his patient's hypnotizability and has used this information to determine a therapeutic course of action.

Once the therapist has determined how hypnotizable the patient is, he can make up a healing ritual and teach it to the patient. Typically, the patient is told, "Hypnotize yourself and do X." In teaching the patient to hypnotize himself, the therapist need only to tell him to do what he did when his suggestibility was assessed. For example, he might be told to stare at a spot on a wall until his eyes close and then get more and more relaxed until he is hypnotized.

It is often a good idea to give the patient a signal which he can use to justify labeling himself as "hypnotized." The therapist might say, "Once your eyes have closed, you will know that you are hypnotized" or "When you are so relaxed that you feel as if you're floating, that's your signal that you have entered the trance state." The therapist can choose such a signal in the same way he devises a placebo communication—by building on the patient's beliefs and experiences. For example, if the patient is capable of a good arm levitation, that can be his signal for the trance state. If not, some other signal can be devised. By observing the patient's response to the initial hypnotic induction and questioning him afterward, it should be easy to find something that the patient can use to tell himself that he is hypnotized.

Once the patient has learned how to hypnotize himself, the therapist can tell him what to suggest to himself while hypnotized. Naturally, the way in which this ritual is explained is extremely important, and the therapist should emphasize the patient's beliefs in telling him why it works. The patient can then practice the healing ritual on his own and cure himself outside therapy. This process of self-cure is illustrated in the case study that follows.

I am presenting this case for several reasons. First, it gives a clear picture of the use of hypnotic healing rituals.

The case is also rather dramatic in that it involves major changes in severe problems in only two sessions. Finally, because the patient was extremely hypnotizable, the case provides an illustration of the way in which her suggestibility relates to both her problems and her treatment. In short, this case study shows the remarkable change possible when extreme suggestibility and the right therapeutic approach are combined.

When Eve T. was admitted to a mental hospital where I worked, the staff members who saw her said that her makeup and coarse manner gave her the appearance of a streetwalker. She was a thirty-six-year–old divorcee who had lived with her two children at the home of her very proper parents for the six years following her divorce. Her parents indicated that she had always been a sweet and gentle "nice girl," quite unlike the way she acted on entering the hospital.

During the week before her admission, Mrs. T.'s ex-husband had made one of his rare visits to see the children and had put on what she referred to as his "loving father act." One evening that week Mrs. T. left her parents' house to visit a friend—and disappeared. After three days of frantic searching, her father located her in the apartment of a "disreputable" man whom she had met at one of the numerous bars she visited. When her father found her, she was quite upset and claimed to have no memory of the events of the previous three days. He then brought her to the hospital, and she agreed to enter voluntarily.

During the first few days of her hospitalization, her behavior changed back rapidly to her previous innocence; and, when I saw her for the first time, there was no trace of coarseness in her appearance.

While in the hospital, she complained of feelings of weakness, migraine headaches, and dizziness, and she fainted several times. In interviews with a psychiatrist and a psychologist, she also admitted to a long history of visual and

80

auditory hallucinations and of delusions of other people "controlling my mind." At the same time, however, there was nothing far-out about either the flow of her speech or her manner of relating to others.

I was called in to interview Mrs. T. in order to clarify the diagnosis and see whether I could do anything therapeutic with her. The issue of diagnosis was in part legitimate because the fainting spells, weakness, headaches, memory disruption, and sudden change in behavior might be the result of some form of brain dysfunction. However, neurological examinations and tests had already ruled out this possibility. The diagnostic issue was really part of the sort of labeling game indulged in all too often in mental hospitals. Was she schizophrenic because of her delusions and hallucinations? Might her fainting spells and other somatic symptoms indicate that she was a conversion hysteric? Perhaps her disappearance and subsequent amnesia meant that she was in a fugue state. Or, wonder of wonders, might her sudden change from saint to sinner mean that she was that rarest of all psychopathological birds, a case of multiple personality? Despite these questions, everyone on the clinical staff knew what Mrs. T. was like; she was as I have described her. Unfortunately, nobody knew what to make of her, so the staff focused their efforts on labeling her. In other words, the diagnostic question was really an attempt to deal with the staff's puzzlement (rather than the patient's problems) by putting Mrs. T. in a familiar mental illness pigeon-hole.

Despite my reservations about the labeling game,[4] I recognized that I could be of help to Mrs. T. only if I

---

[4] In this example I have emphasized only that diagnoses serve the staff's needs while remaining irrelevant to the patient's treatment. Unfortunately, some diagnostic labels (schizophrenia, for example) can also have destructive effects for the rest of a patient's life. Not only does society ostracize those who bear the insignia of deviance, but it also dooms them to live with a self-image of incurable insanity.

worked within the limitations set by the preconditions of therapy. Therefore, even though I was not entirely satisfied with the nature of the referral, I agreed to try both to clarify the diagnosis and to be of therapeutic assistance. Naturally, my intent was to concentrate my efforts on the latter, more important question.

I first met with Mrs. T. about a week after she had been hospitalized. By this time, I already knew a fair amount about her from both other staff members and the hospital records. I began the session by explaining why I was meeting with her, and she seemed eager to cooperate with my efforts to be of assistance. When I asked her to review with me the problems for which she was seeking help at the hospital, she mentioned running away and fainting spells. After briefly discussing these problems with her, I explained that some people with such problems could be helped by the use of hypnosis. When I asked whether she would like to see if hypnosis could help her, she said yes and appeared interested in this new possibility. I then explained that people differ in hypnotizability and that I would have to see how hypnotizable she was to determine whether hypnosis could help her. Her immediate and interested acceptance of everything I said, as well as her willingness—almost eagerness—to follow my suggestion that she be hypnotized, hinted that she would be a good hypnotic subject.

Her behavior after the hypnotic induction was quite dramatic. She responded promptly to all suggestions and had no trouble experiencing the most difficult hypnotic phenomena. Among these were age regression, auditory and visual hallucinations, and negative visual hallucinations (not seeing objects in the room which I suggested she would be unable to see). Finally, after I had given her the signal to cease being hypnotized, she reported "spontaneous amnesia" —that is, she could not remember what had happened during hypnosis.

I was encouraged by the similarity between Mrs. T.'s hypnotic performance (hallucinations and amnesia) and her clinical problems. I therefore explained, in a matter-of-fact way, that she was extremely hypnotizable and that I was going to show her how to use self-hypnosis to deal with her problems. Naturally, she was intrigued by these revelations, and she learned self-hypnosis immediately by following my instructions.

I then asked her to hypnotize herself so that I could tell her how to work with her problems. I had instructed her to use an arm levitation as her signal that she was hypnotized, and in this manner I was able to use her arm as my signal that she was ready to follow my suggestions.

Once her arm was raised, I asked her what problem bothered her most. She said that it was the fainting. I then asked her to imagine vividly that she was in the situation just a few moments before she last fainted and, once the image was clear in her mind, to tell me what it was like. Her face became tense, and she said that she was walking toward the water fountain in the day room of her ward.

I asked her to consider a hundred-point anxiety scale where zero was the calmest she had ever been and one hundred was the most tense. As she imagined herself walking toward the water fountain, I asked her how anxious she felt on that scale. She replied, "Seventy." I then gave her the following instructions: "In other words, you are quite anxious. As you can see, the reason you fainted was that you were very anxious. Fortunately, you are hypnotizable, so you can learn how to relax whenever you get anxious. In this way, you won't have to faint. All you have to do now to relax is say the word *calm* to yourself and imagine that you are getting very relaxed. By doing so, you can relax down to zero very rapidly. Go ahead and try it, and tell me when you're at zero." In a few seconds she smiled and said, "I'm at zero now." "Good," I said. "As you can see, that was very easy.

In the future, any time that you start to get dizzy or very anxious, all you have to do is hypnotize yourself, relax to zero, and come out of the trance. Then you'll be all right."

Next, I told her that when she opened her eyes she would be able to remember what had happened while she was hypnotized and that she could bring herself out of the trance whenever she was ready. She opened her eyes a few seconds later, and we discussed what had just taken place. In talking with her, I emphasized that this technique gave her control over her own behavior. I pointed out that, because she was extremely hypnotizable, she probably went into trances frequently, especially when she was under stress. With this technique, she could use her hypnotizability to achieve her own ends rather than being victimized by it. I also asked her whether she sometimes had experiences in which the world seemed strange or unreal. She said that she did, and I explained that these were times when she was spontaneously going into a trance. All she had to do to stop this experience was to give herself the signal for coming out of the trance (I had told her to count backward from three to one and make a fist). Finally, I suggested that she practice self-hypnosis several times a day until she was used to it and added that she would probably be used to it in a few days.

That was our first session. It took less than an hour, and a tremendous amount was accomplished. Two healing rituals for specific problems were introduced: self-hypnosis and relaxation for fainting spells and the coming-out-of-the-trance signal for feelings of unreality. I transmitted many placebo communications in both my explanations of the healing rituals and my confident, professional manner. Because Mrs. T. was extremely suggestible, I did not need to qualify my confident statements, if something did not work, I knew that she would accept the excuses I later made up. Finally, the new and unusual experiences which she had had in the session (hypnosis, self-hypnosis, and relaxation) served as proof to her that she would be able to change.

Before I met with Mrs. T. a week later (for our second and last session), I made inquiries about whether there had been any changes in her behavior in the ward. The staff reported two new developments: She had not fainted again, and, in contrast to her previous passivity and compliance with any demands made on her, she had become more assertive. She had questioned a number of the hospital's meaningless routines and had become angry with another patient who was continually asking for cigarettes.

With this knowledge in mind, I began the second session by asking Mrs. T. how the previous week had gone. She said that, although she had begun to get dizzy a few times, she had done the self-hypnosis exercise and had not fainted. I tried to trace what had happened in the situations just preceding her getting dizzy, but she was unable to give any clear descriptions. I was left with the impression, however, that she had gotten dizzy in situations where people had been insistent in telling her what to do.

After discussing the events of the previous week, I asked Mrs. T. whether she would like to do something about her other problems—especially those which led her to enter the hospital. When she said that she wanted very much to do so, I asked her to hypnotize herself. Once her arm was raised, I asked her to tell me what had been happening during the time just before she ran away. "My parents and my husband were controlling my mind," she said.[5] "What happened?" I repeated. Mrs. T. explained how her husband, who had done nothing for the children since their divorce, had come for a visit laden with presents. During his stay, he made a point of letting her know what an inadequate mother

[5] People who talk this way easily convince others that they are crazy. And, once others respond to them as if they were crazy, they come to see themselves in the same light. This self-image in turn leads to a vicious circle of more crazy behavior. For this reason, the use of persuasive techniques to modify Mrs. T.'s "delusion" provides a refreshing contrast to the more common, antitherapeutic approach of asking, "When did you first start feeling this way?"

and worthless person she was. She was unable to respond to him angrily and instead began to feel that he might be right. Then, when she spoke to her parents about how upset he had made her, they took his side. They told her that she should be grateful for his presents and his interest in the children. They also said that anything unpleasant he said to her was unimportant and that she should ignore it. It was after these events that she left to visit a friend and indulged in the three days of rebellion which she could not remember.

She seemed quite upset while she told this story, and I noticed that she made a fist (the coming-out-of-the-trance signal) at several points. Taking a cue from this signal, I made the following series of interpretations: "When you said that they controlled your mind, I gather that you were referring to the way in which you believed the bad things they said about you." "Yes." "As you know, you are extremely hypnotizable. What was really happening when you thought they were controlling your mind was that you were going into a trance and following their suggestions. Now you know that, by counting from three to one and making a fist, you can prevent this. You can also make a fist behind your back or somewhere else where they can't see it so they won't know you're resisting them. . . . Of course, when you're trapped in the same house with them, it is kind of hard to prevent everything they say from getting through to you." "It certainly is." "What else could you do?" I asked. "I could move away from home." "That sounds like a good idea." "But they could still control my mind, even at a distance," she said. "How could they do that?" "They could call me on the telephone."

I pointed out that, if the telephone conversation got too difficult for her, she could always hang up. In addition, however, I asked why she did not fight back more. "I'm afraid I might kill them," she said. "You aren't going to kill anyone." "I'm not?"[6] "No. Everyone feels like killing people

[6] This response suggests that even someone as hypnotizable as Mrs.

86

when he's angry with them. It's a natural feeling. And you can use this feeling as a way of knowing that you're angry, so that you can decide what to do. When you feel like killing someone, that's your way of knowing that you're angry at him. For example, if you were in line at a movie theater and someone pushed in front of you, you might feel angry. In fact, if he was really rude, you might even feel like killing him. But once you knew that you were angry you wouldn't actually kill him. Instead, you could say something like 'excuse me. I was here first.' "

Mrs. T. nodded, apparently indicating that she had accepted the suggestions of not worrying about killing people and of becoming more assertive. I therefore mentioned that I had heard she had been standing up for her rights more on the ward. She agreed that she had been, and I praised her for it.

I then asked whether she had any other problems. She said that she was bothered by hallucinations, and I asked her to describe them. She said that she would hear a man's voice behind her, calling her name. When she turned around, she would see the outline of a man, which would rapidly fade away. This hallucination (her only one) had been bothering her periodically for many years.

I asked her to imagine the outline vividly and then to imagine the form of the outline gradually filling in. After a few moments she began to breathe heavily and look very upset. "I can't do it," she said.

I told her to stop imagining it and to relax herself to zero. Then, after she had become relaxed, I asked her to try again. This time, although quite upset, she was able to fill in the man's body. Before filling in the face, she complained that it was too difficult, and I had her stop and relax once

---

T. has difficulty accepting an unjustified suggestion which flies in the face of her strong beliefs. I therefore gave a psychological "explanation" to justify what I said, expecting that her faith in me as a psychologist would allow her to believe the explanation.

more. The third time she was able to fill in the face too. He was an old man whom she did not know, and he was in the basement of her elementary school. Suddenly she cried out that she could not go on and complained of a splitting headache.

I told her to stop imagining the scene and to relax. She did so but said that she still had the headache. I took this as her way of saying that she really did not want to go on, so I said to her, "All right, we won't do that anymore. As far as your headache is concerned, you're fortunate to be so hypnotizable. All you have to do to get rid of pain is to hypnotize yourself—as you already are now—and then imagine that the pain doesn't hurt. Once you do so, the pain will go away. Go ahead and try it." In a few seconds she smiled and said, "The headache is gone."

"Good," I said. "As far as the hallucination of the man is concerned, we can see that it came about when you were anxious. Therefore, if you hypnotize yourself and relax whenever you get really anxious, you will be able to prevent the hallucination. Of course, if it still bothers you, you can always come to see me again, and we can find out all about it." I felt that the threat of making her relive her painful experience with the old man would further motivate her to give up the hallucination.

After this interaction, I asked her whether she had any other problems. She said that she did not. Based on what I had learned about Mrs. T. from both her and other staff members, I was inclined to agree that we had dealt with the core of her problems. I therefore used the remainder of the session to terminate therapy.

First, I reviewed briefly each of Mrs. T.'s problems and the healing ritual she was to use for it. I then suggested that, other than the inevitable reactions to life's ups and downs, she was unlikely to have any further serious problems. If she were to have such a problem, however, I suggested that she would be able to figure out a way to overcome it—by either a new use of self-hypnosis or some other means. Finally, in the unlikely case that she were to develop a problem she could not handle by herself, she could always make an appointment to see me.

After making these suggestions, I told her that, when she came out of the trance, she would be able to remember everything that she was capable of remembering. If there was anything that was too painful to remember, it would stay forgotten at present but would emerge gradually later as she grew capable of tolerating it.

I then asked Mrs. T. to bring herself out of the trance whenever she was ready. She opened her eyes a few seconds later, and we briefly reviewed the ground that we had covered. She remembered everything except the part of the session in which she had filled in the outline of the hallucination. She seemed to feel that her problems had been conquered, and she expressed considerable gratitude as she left. She was discharged from the hospital shortly thereafter.

Several months later, I telephoned Mrs. T. to find out how she was doing. She said that things were going well. Although she still became dizzy occasionally, she had used self-hypnosis effectively and had never fainted. Similarly, she was almost always able to rid herself of headaches; and, on the rare occasions when she had been unable to do away with the pain completely, she had at least been able to diminish it significantly. She was still living with her parents, but she had enrolled in a job training program which she had previously been too timid to attempt. Her plans were to finish the program, get a job, and move out of her parents' house as soon as she was capable of supporting her children.

When I inquired about the outline of a person that had upset her, she stated that something very unusual had happened. For several weeks after she had left the hospital, she had not been bothered by it. Suddenly, one afternoon she saw it again. As she looked at it, the outline filled in, and she saw that it was herself. Then the image went way, and it had not reappeared.

I "explained" to Mrs. T. that sometimes people unconsciously work out their problems by themselves. That the outline had filled in and become herself was probably her unconscious way of telling herself that her troubles were not "out there" but within herself. Now that she had unconsciously achieved this insight, she probably would never be troubled by the image again. Naturally, she agreed that my explanation seemed reasonable and repeated that everything was going well for her. In saying good-by, she again expressed her gratitude for my help; and, in accepting her thanks, I pointed out that she had really done the bulk of the work by her use of the techniques she had learned in therapy.

One might speculate that Mrs. T.'s extreme suggestibility, coupled with years of training in submissive "femininity," led to her inability to cope with demands by significant others that she think or do something against her will. An educated guess about her response to such demands is that she complied in minor matters, attempted to tune people out ("went into a trance") when the issue became more important and the pressure increased, and took extreme action (fainted or ran away) when all else failed. If this guess is accurate, one might further speculate that Mrs. T.'s hallucinations occurred in situations where she was pressured to think or act against her will. In other words, it is possible that such pressure made her feel as she had with the dirty old man in her elementary school basement.

However, the effectiveness of therapy with Mrs. T. was not dependent on the total accuracy of such speculations. Instead, the decisive therapeutic factors were that she was given a new and believable way of thinking about her problems and a number of concrete things to do about them.

Her vices (symptoms of mental illness) became virtues (proof of her hypnotic ability), and her feeling of being at the mercy of her problems was replaced by a new ability to cure herself.

SEVEN

~~~~~~~~~~~~~~~~~~~~~~~~~~~~~~~~~~~

Applications to Behavior Modification

~~~~~~~~~~~~~~~~~~~~~~~~~~~~~~~~~~~

One of the most exciting recent trends in psychotherapy has been the burgeoning of the field of behavior modification. Behavior modifiers have used experimentally validated principles of psychology in developing new ways of helping people. In a few short years, they have generated many novel therapeutic techniques, and extensive experimental investigation has already demonstrated the effectiveness of several.

Because these techniques involve a direct treatment of the patient's problems, they can easily be made to function as healing rituals; and any beneficial effects of such rituals enhance the patient's expectations of being helped. This increase in faith leads in turn to further improvement.

As was the case with hypnotherapy, the following discussion of certain techniques of behavior modification is quite brief. These techniques have received extensive treatment elsewhere;[1] and the aim of this chapter is restricted to showing how they can be used within the context of placebo therapy.

Systematic desensitization was originally developed as a treatment for phobias, although it has subsequently been used to treat a wide variety of related problems. In brief, when systematic desensitization is used as a treatment technique, the following sequence of events takes place between therapist and patient: (1) The phobic area is identified (for example, fear of heights). (2) Situational dimensions of the phobia are identified (the higher the patient is, the more anxious he becomes). (3) The therapist explains how systematic desensitization works. (4) A graded series of scenes, or hierarchy, is constructed along the phobic dimension, from scenes which disturb the patient least through those which disturb him most (looking out a second floor window, looking out a third floor window . . . through looking down at the street from the top of the Empire State Building). (5) The patient is taught to become deeply relaxed. (6) The phobia is desensitized: While the patient is deeply relaxed, he visualizes the least disturbing scene in the hierarchy until it no longer bothers him. He then visualizes the next-most-disturbing scene until it too no longer makes him anxious. He continues in this manner until even the last scene of the hierarchy is no longer upsetting. When systematic desensitization works, which it does remarkably often, improvement in the patient's real life situation parallels his mastery of the

[1] Suggested readings in behavior modification are included in the Annotated Bibliography.

hierarchy scenes (he is actually able to look down from the roof of a tall building).

A number of hypotheses, predominantly from the field of learning theory, have been advanced to explain why systematic desensitization works. The most prominent hypothesis is the principle of reciprocal inhibition. A therapist explaining how systematic desensitization works in terms of reciprocal inhibition would tell his patient something like the following: "It's impossible to respond to a single stimulus with two incompatible responses. For example, you can't be both tense and relaxed at the same time. Whenever there are two competing responses, a person makes whichever response is stronger. This is how systematic desensitization works. When you are deeply relaxed, your relaxation response is strong. On the other hand, when you imagine looking out a second floor window, your response of tension or anxiety is weak. In this way, the relaxation response reciprocally inhibits, or gets rid of, that small amount of anxiety. In other words, instead of leading to a response of tension, the same stimulus of looking out a second floor window now leads to the new response of relaxation. Thus, your total fear of heights is decreased by a small amount; and the thought of looking out a third floor window bothers you only as much as the thought of looking out a second floor window did previously. By always keeping your relaxation response stronger than your anxiety response, systematic desensitization allows you to get rid of your fear in a deliberate manner."

Other explanations of why systematic desensitization works include extinction (repeated exposure to the fear-producing situation with no bad consequences for the patient) as well as the possibility that the technique is no more than a very scientific-sounding placebo. Regardless of why systematic desensitization works, the explanation functions essentially as a placebo communication. Thus, the therapeutic effect of the explanation must be judged independently of the technique itself.

In considering such an explanation, one might wonder why a behavior modifier would present a patient with so complex and scientific-sounding a rationale. From the point of view of placebo therapy, the best reason is that an assessment of the patient's beliefs suggested that he would be likely to believe such an explanation. Unfortunately, this reason frequently is not the basis for the explanation. Therapy takes place between two believers, and behavior modification is no exception to this rule. The reason behavior modifiers use systematic desensitization is that they believe it works. And, when they explain it to their patients in terms of reciprocal inhibition, they do so because, in all naiveté, they believe the explanation is true.

If, by coincidence, a particular patient finds such a rationale congenial to his beliefs, his therapist has done no harm by his unreflective choice of words. If, however, the patient finds the explanation repugnant to his world view, his therapist has done him a great disservice. By allowing the success of therapy to hinge on the weakening or destruction of a patient's cherished beliefs, the therapist has greatly diminished the chances of success of systematic desensitization.

An objection of other therapists to behavior modification is that conditioning techniques, such as systematic desensitization, teach the patient that he is a dehumanized machine. This argument seems fatuous to me because a person's belief that he is or is not a machine is unlikely to be changed by a brief explanation of a therapeutic technique. However, even though I am unimpressed by the feeling of some therapists that behavior modification techniques are intrinsically dehumanizing, the possibility that a given patient might see them in this light causes me real concern. It is for this reason that explanations of therapeutic techniques should be based on the patient's beliefs rather than on the

95

therapist's theoretical preferences. Unfortunately, this does not seem to be standard practice in behavior modification, and a patient may come along who does not like the behavior modifier's rationale. For example, consider an interaction where the therapist has just finished explaining, in terms of reciprocal inhibition, how he plans to use systematic desensitization to combat his patient's fear of heights. Patient: "That sounds like you're going to try to condition me, like *1984*." Therapist: "Systematic desensitization is nothing like *1984*. It's a technique to get rid of your fear. I thought that's why you came to see me in the first place." Patient: "Yes, but I didn't want to be conditioned!" Therapist: "I'm sorry you feel like that, but as a therapist I have to recommend the treatment that's best in my judgment." Therapy is then terminated, and the therapist attributes his loss of a patient to insufficient motivation or perhaps to creeping Freudianism.

It is, of course, possible in this example that any explanation of systematic desensitization would have been unacceptable to the patient. Sometimes the medium really is the message; that is, a given technique may be so at variance with a patient's world view or conception of therapy that there is no way of getting him to accept it. And, if a therapist can find no mutually acceptable alternative course of action, therapy may still have to be terminated at the outset.

Although the above result might have been unavoidable, such a conclusion is by no means certain, for a different explanation of systematic desensitization might well have succeeded. Thus, it was the therapist's lack of foresight in offering an explanation without first considering its meaning to the patient which precluded the exploration of alternatives.

Once a therapist has accepted the notion of basing his explanations on his patients' beliefs rather than on truth, such explanations are not difficult to formulate. The following brief examples give two explanations of systematic desensitization which differ widely because they were given to two very different people.

An engineer who had a phobia seemed to hold a rather mechanistic view of both the world and himself. He was quite organized in his presentation of why he was seeking therapy, and my impression was that he would be attracted to an efficient and scientific form of therapy. In explaining the use of the systematic desensitization to treat his phobia, I therefore gave a miniature lecture on the technique along the lines of the above reciprocal inhibition explanation. However, my presentation was more technical, and I even drew a graph to illustrate some of the research findings. He appeared impressed by both the logic of the technique and the respect for his intelligence which my explanation implied.

Although the engineer was just the sort of person who is receptive to the standard rationale given for systematic desensitization, a young man who consulted me in a university counseling center was quite the opposite. He had long hair and was bearded, beaded, and bedecked in the most colorful hippie tradition. He too had a phobia, but his entire life style suggested that he would be turned off by a conditioning rationale for systematic desensitization. His concern with consciousness expansion, which included an eagerness to experience new sensations, seemed the opposite of the environmental and mechanistic emphases of systematic desensitization. At the same time, I thought that he would be equally unenthusiastic about the more traditional therapeutic approach of ignoring his phobia and instead directing his attention to increasing his understanding of himself. Because his phobia was "where he was at" and because he was more interested in nonverbal sensations than in talking, it seemed to me that he would find such an approach to be both unspontaneous and intellectualized.

I gave him the following explanation—which proved successful—for systematic desensitization: "I think I know a way that would enable you to deal with your fear fairly rapidly, but it would involve your experiencing some hypnoticlike phenomena. Would you be willing to consider such a possibility? [Naturally, he agreed.] The approach I have in mind involves your learning to achieve a semihypnotic state of relaxation. Once you were in this state, I would help you little by little to experience your fear, confront it, and eventually overcome it. By lowering your conscious defenses, the state of relaxation would enable you to experience your feelings more fully and in this way overcome your fear by becoming totally aware of it."

The phobias of both patients were successfully desensitized; and I believe that the explanations of systematic desensitization were an important factor. A scientific explanation increased the engineer's motivation for treatment and enabled him to benefit from the placebo effect as well as from systematic desensitization itself. The explanation to the hippie in terms of an altered state of consciousness allowed him to derive the same motivational and therapeutic benefits.

Hopefully, as increasing numbers of therapists make use of systematic desensitization in their practice, they too will base their explanations on their patients' beliefs. Furthermore, the wide range of other behavior modification techniques explained before use are all open to differing explanations, depending on the beliefs of the patient involved. Thus, a therapist being trained in behavior modification techniques should receive simultaneous training in making placebo explanations. For example, if a supervisor role-plays a variety of patients who are being told about a given technique (for example, a truck driver, a kindergarten teacher, and a religious fanatic), a therapist can gain valuable practice in explaining the same healing ritual to patients with widely differing beliefs.

As already mentioned, the validity of some behavior

modification techniques has been demonstrated above and beyond the placebo effect. Paradoxically, the existence of such valid techniques makes possible a simple strategy for enhancing the placebo effect itself. In brief, this strategy involves using a valid technique to achieve a rapid cure of a minor problem. Once this cure has been effected, its success can be used as a way of mobilizing the patient's faith to deal with more difficult problems. In other words, the main reason for treating the minor problem first (or at all in some cases) is to maximize the placebo effect and hence the chance of success in treating a truly difficult problem. The following description of part of the treatment of a complex case should provide a useful illustration of this strategy.

When Mrs. P. came to a clinic where I was working to seek help for her nine-year-old son, Bird P., she was rather pessimistic. She said that, though she doubted that therapy could help her "brain damaged" boy, she wanted to leave no stone unturned in seeking help for him. When I asked her what his problems were, she focused mainly on his hyperactivity—which is frequently a symptom of brain damage. As she described this hyperactivity further, it appeared to involve calling out and otherwise disrupting his school class as well as running around a lot and concocting attention-getting mischief at home. She also said that she was concerned about his work in arithmetic. For two years, Bird had been unable to learn the multiplication table. During this time, Mrs. P. had practiced with him after school daily and had even enrolled him in summer school—all to no avail. Furthermore, because of his disciplinary problem and poor schoolwork, his teacher had told Mrs. P. that he was in danger of being kept in the same grade. Mrs. P. and I discussed some of his other problems, which were also dealt with in the course of treatment, but they are not relevant to this presentation.

At the end of the interview, I told Mrs. P. that I would be willing to see her son and contact the other professionals involved in his case to determine whether therapy might be of help to Bird. If it did seem possible that therapy could help him, I said that I would be glad to work with him. For her part, Mrs. P. assured me that she would be ready to participate in his treatment in any way I might request.

Once we had established this preliminary contact (that is, to investigate whether or not to enter into a therapeutic contract), I began an extensive assessment. During this time, in addition to meeting again with Mrs. P., I interviewed Bird, gave him several psychological tests, observed him in class, and consulted with his teacher, pediatrician, and pediatric neurologist. The following is a brief summary of what I learned.

Mrs. P. was a warm, likable woman and a patient and sympathetic mother. As a consequence, her three other children were developing beautifully, and their smooth development made Bird's difficulties even more noticeable. Naturally, Mrs. P. had devoted much extra time and energy to trying to help him, but her repeated failures as well as her belief that Bird was neurologically impaired had led her to despair of doing anything for him.

At school, his teacher was a rather prim woman who, though clearly concerned about her students, seemed to expect rather more silence and self-control from them than is typical these days. In speaking with her, therefore, I kept in mind the possibility that Bird's behavior might appear more outlandish to her than to a less demanding teacher.

In describing his behavior, Bird's teacher complained that he constantly squirmed in his seat and frequently disrupted the class by calling out or making rude noises. He seemed bent on getting attention and would try almost anything to achieve it. Thus, he had recently jumped out of his seat, pulled forward his shirt pockets in imitation of breasts, and wiggled his hips, to the uproarious delight of his classmates. Like his mother, Bird's teacher felt defeated; everything she had done to get him to change had failed.

When I sat in the back of his class one afternoon to observe him in action, his "hyperactivity" was absent. He did not call out or disrupt the class in any way; and, though he occasionally squirmed in his seat, so did his classmates. After class, his teacher seemed embarrassed that he had not performed as expected. I told her that such occurrences were not unusual and that it had been valuable for me to observe him in the class setting. Even though his teacher was upset by his quietude, I was privately impressed by Bird's ability to control his behavior merely because of my presence—a very unusual kind of brain damage.

During my first interview alone with Bird, he seemed tense for the first few minutes. I assume that the reason was that I was a stranger and the interview situation was unusual for him because he quickly warmed up to me and talked freely thereafter. He cooperated fully in taking a number of tests, and he generally relished the one-to-one attention I gave him. In fact, his teacher told me that before my visit he had boasted to his classmates that I was coming especially to see him. As I got to know Bird better, it became increasingly evident that he greatly desired the approval or at least the attention of others. The attention of adults was more rewarding for Bird than that of his peers, and his mother's attention was the most highly prized of all.

Bird's performance on the psychological tests indicated that he was of average intelligence. In fact, the most striking characteristic of his test results was that he performed well on tasks where he should have had difficulties. He was above average in his ability to do arithmetic problems in his head(!) and gave no evidence of the kinds of perceptual or motor difficulties often associated with brain damage.

The reports which I received from Bird's pediatrician and pediatric neurologist were of great interest in rounding

101

out my understanding of his problems. Apparently, Bird had had two convulsions of unknown origin, both during his sleep. The first had been when he was three and a half years old, and the second was at the age of five. His EEGs had indicated the possibility of some brain damage—although children's EEGs are known to be unreliable diagnostic instruments (the EEG, together with other tests of brain dysfunction, is more valid for older patients). At the same time, however, Bird had never shown any abnormality in his neurological examinations. Although the neurologist had been willing to make the word-game diagnosis of idiopathic epilepsy (convulsions of unknown origin), he doubted that Bird had any organic deficit; and he even went so far as to suggest that Bird's school and home problems were probably of emotional origin. However, despite the likelihood that Bird had no neurological damage, his physicians recognized that they could not definitely rule out the possibility. They therefore decided to place him on a low dosage of medication to prevent his having another seizure just in case the previous two had been of organic origin.

Based on these reports, it seemed likely that Bird's physicians had inadvertently communicated to his mother something other than their findings. Mrs. P. had probably assembled in her mind the following three pieces of information: The doctors said that brain damage could not be ruled out; they prescribed medication for him; and my other children are developing fine, but nothing I do seems to help Bird. I speculated that she had concluded, "Bird's problems are the result of brain damage. The doctors probably don't want to say so because they don't want to upset me or because they are scientific and wouldn't say such a thing unless they were absolutely certain."

Given all this information, it seemed unlikely that Bird had brain damage; and, even if he did, it was probably irrelevant to his problems or their treatment. However, his mother's belief that he did have brain damage, as well as

102

her belief that he could not be helped (which was shared by his teacher), seemed to be critical obstructions to the success of therapy. I therefore decided to work with Bird in therapy on the basis of a diagnostic formulation discussed below. Furthermore, in beginning treatment, I decided to use the strategy of success to gain the optimistic cooperation of both his teacher and his mother.

Operant conditioning is the brainchild of B. F. Skinner. Briefly stated, his theory views behavior as a function of its environmental consequences.[2] Thus, behavior which is followed by rewarding consequences increases in frequency (is conditioned), while behavior which is followed by no consequences—neither reward nor punishment—decreases in frequency (is extinguished). Attention has been shown to be an important reward (or reinforcer) for children—as was clear with Bird—and is effective in increasing the frequency of behavior which it follows. Unfortunately, attention sometimes has the paradoxical effect of increasing just that behavior which a parent would like to decrease. For example, a parent who says, "Stand up straight!" every time his child slouches is actually training his child to have bad posture because the parent's attention follows the child's poor posture and thereby makes it worse. According to Skinner, the proper way for a parent to teach his child good posture is to ignore slouching, thereby diminishing its frequency, and to say, "You look good standing up straight like that!" when his child's posture is good.

I assumed that an unfortunate paradoxical effect, similar to that in the bad posture example, was responsible for Bird's problems. Thus, although Mrs. P. had done an excellent job of raising her other children, Bird's convulsions had likely led her to treat him differently; that is, as the result of an understandable motherly concern, she might well have remained alert for any sign of abnormality in Bird's

[2] Readings on operant conditioning are included among the readings on behavior modification in the Annotated Bibliography.

behavior and rushed to shower attention on him when he seemed upset or acted up. She might have ignored as unimportant such behavior in her other children and thereby decreased its frequency, but attending to the same behavior in Bird would have had the opposite effect. And the reason that Bird had not mastered the multiplication table was probably that he was receiving considerable attention from both his mother and his teacher as a reward for not learning it.

Because the multiplication table was a small and easily accessible problem, I decided to make it the initial focus of the strategy of success. I began by testing Bird on his knowledge of multiplication and found that he already knew more than half of the table. In addition, many of the combinations which he did not know were mirror image pairs (for example, six times seven and seven times six), thus diminishing further the area of his ignorance. For Bird to learn this small part of the multiplication table, someone had only to reward him for correct answers and ignore wrong ones. I therefore devised a game for him to play with his mother in which she gave him one point for each correct answer and a penny for every ten points he earned. Mrs. P. and Bird agreed to play this game every day for ten or fifteen minutes.

When I saw Mrs. P. in our session a week later, she reported in amazement that Bird had mastered the entire multiplication table. She was delighted with this development because she had only dared to hope for a slight improvement in so short a time. She said that Bird was pleased to have mastered the table at last and that his teacher was also happily surprised by the change.

Riding the crest of the new optimism about Bird's potential for change, I immediately initiated treatment of his more pervasive problem of hyperactivity. I explained to Mrs. P. how she could help Bird to calm down at home by altering her pattern of responding to him (that is, by attending to him in his quieter moments and ignoring him when he was acting up). I also planned with his teacher a program of rewards (gold stars) which he would receive for staying in his seat and not calling out for successively longer periods. By taking the stars home, Bird would be able to supplement his teacher's praise for his good behavior with praise and attention from his mother. (If the praise and attention had not been enough to change Bird's behavior, I would have set up a system in which he could have traded stars for prizes, but prizes proved unnecessary.)

Over a period of several weeks, this program was quite successful. Because his first response to his mother's and teacher's new behavior was an exaggeration of his habitual attention-getting ploys (a Skinnerian would call this reaction an extinction burst), it was quite difficult for them to ignore him. However, because they had been warned of this possibility and because of the hope engendered by Bird's mastery of the multiplication table, they were able to stand firm and reward only improved behavior with their attention. Their conscientiousness in turn enabled the program to succeed.

As Bird changed in these areas as well as in others not discussed here, he seemed to gain self-confidence. My guess is that, as the result of changes in him and in people important to him, he felt more in control of himself. Thus, his "hyperactive" behavior seemed to be out of control (although a Skinnerian would say that is was "controlled" by its consequences in the same way as his newer, tame behavior). Not only did he view himself in this way but he could see that his mother and teacher also believed that he was out of control. Once he saw that he could regulate his own behavior and that others were aware of his change, it was natural for his self-esteem to increase.

My entire involvement with Bird's case lasted just over four months—nine sessions with Mrs. P., during several of which Bird was present for part of the time, four sessions alone with Bird, and two school visits. As indicated above, most of my work was involved in assessment, so the treatment phase was actually quite brief. However, the changes in Bird's behavior during treatment were dramatic, and word from another teacher in his school several months later indicated that they had continued after termination.

I have included this case fragment to illustrate the strategy of success as an application of placebo principles to behavior modification. Because some skeptics may not see a great resemblance between my treatment of Bird P. and faith-healing, I feel compelled to relate what Mrs. P. said to me near the end of our last session: "I prayed to God to help me with my son, and I feel that you were the answer to my prayers."

In thanking her for these generous words, I naturally emphasized that it was she who had helped Bird by changing her behavior and that I had merely given her a few clues on what to do. I attributed Bird's change to what she had done to encourage her to continue in her new behavior; the way she acted was crucial to maintaining Bird's improvement. At the same time, however, her religious reference helped to emphasize for me the essential similarity of the curative powers of faith in both psychotherapy and religious healing.

EIGHT

Applications to Group Therapy

Over the past decade, many novel forms of group interaction have appeared and have rapidly attracted vast numbers of adherents. People are now spending millions of dollars for an opportunity to scream at the top of their lungs or to embrace people whom they have never met before and will never meet again. When the participants claim that they have found new meaning in their lives as a result of engaging in these and similar activities, it is reasonable to ask whether the processes of placebo therapy might not be responsible for their miraculous transformations.

Part of this flowering of human relations groups has been the invention of many new techniques designed to achieve specific ends. For example, screaming or shouting is supposed to release pent-up hostility, while looking into the eyes of another group member should increase one's capacity for intimacy. In contrast with the data already supporting some of the techniques of behavior modification, there is no experimental evidence to demonstrate whether the new group techniques achieve their stated ends above and beyond the placebo effect. In the absence of such evidence, I can only report my personal judgment of these techniques and their relationship to the placebo principles thus far discussed. (I should mention that I have both experienced the techniques as a member of groups in which they were used and experimented with them in groups that I have led.)

In evaluating the so-called "touchie-feelie" techniques, I must admit that they do provide amusement and occasionally even intense emotional experiences for many people, although a few individuals are deeply upset by them. Despite such emotional reactions, however, I feel that the techniques serve primarily as healing rituals and that they have little or no therapeutic value beyond the placebo effect. In other words, my view is that, when the techniques achieve their stated ends, they do so because the group members believe that they work, not because they are actually valid. The rationales for the techniques are believable; they are either explicitly explained by the group leader or have been disseminated to the members by friends, books, or the mass media; and the members of the group wish to achieve the ends toward which the techniques are aimed. Such a combination of factors makes for effective healing rituals.

Let us consider a typical group technique: falling backward. This technique, which is aimed at developing the sense of trust, works as follows. A member of the group stands up straight while another member stands a few feet behind him, ready to catch him. At the leader's suggestion, the designated member begins to sway backward. When he starts to fall, but after the point where he could brace himself to stop falling, the person behind him catches him.

As a result of participating in this technique, the "fall-guy" is supposed to have his trust in his fellow man vindicated and to feel even more confident that he will not be "let down" if he risks himself with his neighbor. Should a participant be so untrusting as to break his fall by putting one foot behind him, he is encouraged to try again, so that he can learn that people are more willing to "back him up" than he imagines.

It is easy to see that falling backward is an excellent healing ritual. The explanation about the sense of trust is a believable one; and when someone who was at first unable to fall backward succeeds in doing so, he can see that he has changed. This knowledge in turn makes it easy for him to believe that he has become a more trusting person.

However, a striking fact about the technique is that, for years, falling backward has been one of the most common hypnotic inductions. The hypnotist stands behind the subject while suggesting that he sway back farther and farther. Then, when the subject falls and is caught by the hypnotist, instead of being told, "Now you are more trusting," he is told, "Now you are hypnotized." Among the thousands of people who have been hypnotized by this induction, I know of no reports of anyone's sense of trust suddenly increasing. The absence of such reports suggests that any effect on the sense of trust which comes from falling backward is due to the placebo effect rather than to the effect of the technique itself. And, until there is experimental evidence to the contrary, this line of thinking is what leads me to be skeptical of the theoretical rationales for similar techniques as well.

Given people's emotional reactions to the techniques, there must be something more to them than the placebo effect. I have indicated that I do not believe that the "something extra" is validity; I think that the additional element is just what it appears to be—emotional excitement. The techniques involve sensory pleasure, hints of erotic possibilities, novelty, emotional play, and the status of engaging in the newest, hottest item on the therapy market.

These qualities were well illustrated in a marathon that I participated in as a group member a few years ago. All the participants were eager to try out the many techniques which they had either heard of or had actually experienced in other settings. Despite the stated purpose of the group, which was to learn about ourselves and about group process, a vocal minority of the group kept after the leader to stop all the talk and get on with the techniques. These people were more interested in the excitement of the techniques themselves than in achieving the goals of the group. This interest was particularly evident during breaks for meals, when nearly all the participants went off in pairs or small groups to try out various techniques with one another. When the leader finally got around to using the techniques in the formal group setting, I thought he did so partially in order for us to get them out of our systems so that we could return to the business of the group.

While all this was going on, it was also clear that a status hierarchy had emerged among the group members which differentiated among us according to the amount of group experience we had had. People at the top of the hierarchy had participated in many groups, knew all the techniques, and might even have had experience in leading groups. They knew how to have an insight, how to be absorbed by a technique, how to express emotions, and how to be sensitive (for example, "I sense an inner beauty in you which moves me deeply"). People at the bottom of the hierarchy were enjoying their first group experience and were eager to learn from their more sophisticated peers. The novices rapidly learned to stop being defensive ("I think that tomorrow is Wednesday") and open themselves to new emotions ("I feel that tomorrow is Wednesday").

Just as the excitement, intimacy, and prestige of

110

these new techniques appear to me to be responsible for most people's positive emotional reactions to them, I believe that they also account for the occasional negative emotional reactions. Some people are too threatened by intimacy and the unknown to cooperate in trying out the techniques. As they refuse to give in to other members' urgings and express doubts about the group mystique, they are at first attacked for being defensive and then ostracized. Although such people typically refrain from joining groups, participants do join for many reasons and with diverse expectations. Thus, it is not surprising that an occasional person's experience consists of joining a group where the other members not only seem eager to do bizarre things but also attack him and force him to leave when he questions what they are doing. Such an experience is clearly a disturbing one and was in fact responsible for the departure of one of the members from the marathon mentioned above.

I have dwelt on these techniques because they have been the subject of much current interest among group therapists, although I believe that the techniques can be adequately accounted for in terms already discussed and that they have nothing new to contribute to an understanding of placebo therapy. In contrast, other features of group interaction do seem to merit closer attention. The following discussion is devoted to a consideration of these features in various kinds of groups (including those which employ "touchie-feelie" techniques) and of their relationship to the processes involved in faith-healing.

In our culture, religious faith-healing has traditionally been performed in groups because the group setting offers certain unique advantages. Although the manifest goal of faith-healing is to cure the ill, group meetings serve the equally important latent function of converting doubters into believers and strengthening the faith of wavering mem-

111

bers. In other words, one-to-one faith-healing might accomplish just as much curing as group faith-healing,[1] but it would leave unattended the latent function of proselytism.

Group faith-healing achieves this end in several ways. First, the dramatic display of healing and the charismatic leadership of the healer are inspirations for religious conversion or a reaffirmation of faith. Then, the active and public participation in prayer by the group members strengthens their faith; they would appear hypocritical to themselves and those around them if they were merely going through the motions. Furthermore, the belief that it was his prayer which helped to cure his fellow man provides a very personal answer to any spiritual doubts which might trouble a member of the group. Finally, the excitement of the meeting and the evident faith of those around him can serve to reassure a wavering soul (that is, he can tell himself, "If all these other people are such ardent believers, they must be right").

In an important sense, the personal transformation of psychotherapy resembles that of religious conversion. Both the patient with problems and the troubled sinner are dissatisfied with their ways of life and disillusioned with the beliefs on which they are based. These feelings make them ripe for conversion to attractive alternative sets of beliefs and the new ways of life which accompany them.

Because the group setting offers a number of advantages for religious faith-healing, it is not surprising that similar opportunities are present in both group therapy and other secular groups. The magical aura surrounding the

[1] This statement assumes that God is the active agent in faith-healing. Of course, if social forces, such as those of placebo therapy, are responsible for the cure, the group does serve an important function. If the "patient" is cured or at least declares himself cured, he earns a moment of glory among his fellow believers. If, however, he states that he is not cured, he must face at least the shame of being a failure in his spiritual performance and possibly even accusations by himself and others that God refused to cure him because he is undeserving.

therapist's role and the power associated with his position of leadership add to his effectiveness as an instrument of change. Group pressures, especially those initiated or amplified by the leader, also serve as a potent force for changing the beliefs and behavior of individual members. Finally, because the structure of many groups includes contact between members outside group meetings, these pressures can continue to operate tenaciously in the members' everyday lives.

The wide and expanding variety of groups currently in existence makes it impossible to consider in detail the specific ways in which such group forces operate in every different setting. However, the following discussion of the variations in group goals, group structure, and group process should point up some of the aspects of placebo therapy abounding in group interaction.[2]

Group Goals. Every group has a set of goals which defines its purpose and serves as a standard against which progress can be measured. Whether the goals are explicitly stated and agreed upon or poorly defined and left for members to infer, their existence affects everything that takes place within the group. In fact, one of the major sources of difficulty in groups is an implicit conflict among members over the nature of the group's goals. Once this conflict becomes explicit (through the leader's intervention or otherwise), rapid change often takes place. The members might all subscribe to more clearly defined goals, a few members might leave,[3] or the group might dissolve after finding that major differences an irreconcilable.

Although the goals of work groups are relatively

[2] A few references on different types of groups appear in the Annotated Bibliography; and interested readers have no difficulty in applying the concepts of this book to any particular type of group.

[3] Some people who "behave inappropriately" in groups turn out merely to have been in the wrong place. Once they see that the group's goals are not theirs, they can leave and seek fulfillment elsewhere.

clear-cut (the production of goods or services[4]), the goals of other groups are often both less precise and more complex. These goals consist of converting members to new beliefs and behavior. Even though such goals may involve a relatively small part of the members' lives (giving up smoking, for example), goals are typically aimed at a wider area of influence. Clearly, a group's structure should facilitate the attainment of its goals. Thus, the more ambitious its goals, the more a group should be designed to have a broad impact on its members' lives. The following comments should further clarify these interrelationships between group goals and group structure.

Group Structure. A useful way of classifying groups is according to the extent to which they intrude upon their members' lives. Thus, groups might be roughly divided into the categories of total environment; social network; open-ended, limited contact; and fixed duration, limited contact.

Synanon is a good illustration of a *total environment* at work. It is a self-help group made up primarily of heroin addicts whom it houses and employs. The junkie who comes to Synanon personifies the down-and-out sinner seeking salvation. Typically, he has lost the support of friends and family after betraying them to get money for drugs. Not only is he a social outcast but, through his degradation, he has also come to view himself in a wretched light. He has lost faith in his fellow man, justice, the church, and any other ideals he once held. Beyond the oblivion offered by drugs, the only available sources of social gratification are self-destructive ones: the unstable friendship of other addicts and pushers and the excitement of playing cops and robbers. He knows that he is likely to die soon either from an overdose of drugs or as the result of his criminal activities.

---

[4] I do not mean to imply that the ways in which work groups strive to achieve these ends are as straightforward as the goals themselves. Bureaucratic infighting and the mindless drive of organizations toward self-perpetuation point clearly in the other direction.

When Synanon proposes a goal of keeping its members permanently off drugs, the organization must clearly change virtually every aspect of their lives. The addict must renounce not only drugs but the entire environment from which he came. Friends within Synanon must replace those from the drug world, and a new philosophy of life—based on Ralph Waldo Emerson's essay "Self-Reliance"—must replace his embittered cynicism. Further education or job training may be indicated to provide him with the skills necessary to stay out of trouble.

Because Synanon's goals imply the necessity of affecting every aspect of its members' lives, the group must be structured so as to allow unlimited access to their moment-to-moment existence. This is the reason that addicts are both housed and employed by the organization. The emotionally explosive form of group therapy (called the Synanon Game) which occupies many hours of each addict's week is structured so as to maintain the organization's impact on the totality of his environment. Each Game's membership, of roughly ten to fifteen people, includes a cross-section of the people at Synanon. Because no two Games (that is, no two group meetings) have the same membership, the only group to which the members develop an allegiance is the larger organization. During the Game, when attention is focused on an individual member, one important role of the others present is to serve as informants about any shortcomings in his day-to-day life. As these shortcomings are revealed, the other members unite in a vigorous and self-righteous condemnation of such behavior and extract promises of change from their perpetrator. For example, it might be revealed that, while working as an attendant at the Synanon gas station, a member of the group insulted an impatient motorist. He might then be attacked for alienating customers, thereby diminishing the organization's income so that it can no longer support the addicts in the Game with him, causing them to return to the streets and certain death. When he

115

admits culpability, he might be required to promise never to insult customers and to carefully observe and imitate the behavior of a particular experienced attendant who works with him. Subsequently, people from the gas station and from the present Game would check up on his new behavior in future Games.

In addition to this kind of moment-to-moment influence over its members' lives, Synanon also offers a set of beliefs which provides a basis for ultimate self-regulation. These beliefs constitute a secular religion composed of Emerson's essay "Self-Reliance" (its Bible), the wisdom and personal example of Charles Dederich, an ex-alcoholic who founded Synanon (its high priest), and the lives of several addicts who were cured by Synanon and went on to become high officials of the organization (its apostles).

In contrast with Synanon, Alcoholics Anonymous constitutes a *social network*. It too recognizes the utility of a powerful set of beliefs in enabling its members to stay away from liquor. However, instead of Emerson, it offers its members a stiff shot of oldtime religion. Although the content of the beliefs is different, their therapeutic function is the same (naturally, if a particular individual is turned off by Emerson or God, he would be more likely to leave the organization and thereby lose out on its potent therapy).

In a similar way, group pressures operate effectively within A.A. to keep its members dry. Public confessions of their sins as alcoholics and commitments never to drink again put the members in a social position where staying away from alcohol is strongly rewarded and drinking is bitterly condemned. That the approval and disapproval come from a peer group with whom each alcoholic identifies makes these social pressures even more effective Furthermore, because A.A. groups exist all over the United States and because the organization maintains contact with each member —both by word of mouth from other members and through such publications as the *A.A. Grapevine*—it is difficult for members to drift away from its influence and back to alcohol. This type of group structure has a considerably broader impact on its members' lives than do most forms of group therapy. However, A.A. neither houses nor employs its members, so it cannot have the moment-to-moment influence on them which is possible in a total environment such as Synanon.

The structural differences between a total environment and a social network clearly have therapeutic implications for their respective members. For example, a hard core alcoholic who dropped out of A.A. would probably stand a good chance of being cured by Synanon. The reasoning behind this conclusion is that, because some alcoholics have ruined virtually every aspect of their lives (that is, they have lost family, job, and hope), a social network cannot cope with all their problems. By contrast, a total environment offers the pervasive impact on its members' lives which is a prerequisite for success.[5] Such implications emphasize the close interdependence between therapeutic goals and group structure.

Unlike Synanon and A.A., most group therapy takes place within the structure of an *open-ended, limited contact group*. That is, the length and frequency of meetings is fixed, but the total number of meetings is left open—and it is understood that the group may go on for years. The membership of the group is reasonably stable, and, typically, the members do not know each other before the first meeting. Finally if contacts between members outside the group are not actively discouraged, they are at least rare.

The set of beliefs which any particular therapy group

[5] Because heroin is illegal and therefore expensive, addicts are driven to criminal activities to support their habit. Their resultant experiences with prison and the underworld socialize them into the criminal role—making it necessary for therapy to affect all aspects of their lives. If this sequence were not the norm, many noncriminal addicts might, after completing withdrawal from heroin, be kept off drugs by a social network similar to Alcoholics Anonymous.

117

offers its members is usually quite clear in the therapist's[6] mind. Unfortunately, however, unlike Synanon and Alcoholics Anonymous, most therapists do not make their beliefs clear to members at the outset. In fact, one likely reason that most group therapy lasts so long is that it is difficult for the members to guess what the therapist wants them to believe.

The beliefs which any group therapist transmits to his patients are largely determined by his theoretical orientation. Consider, for example, a psychoanalyst's belief that it is good for people to express feelings of anger in their everyday lives so as to avoid the depressive or psychosomatic consequences of anger turned inward. The analyst does not view this as a belief which, if adopted by group members, would help them to change their behavior (that is, if they believed it, they would be more likely to express anger). He regards it as a fact. Because it is a fact in his eyes, he has no particular reason to tell it to his patients—any more than he would tell them that two plus two is four. Furthermore, his decision not to mention it is based on other psychoanalytic "facts" which indicate that revealing as little as possible about himself or his beliefs is most therapeutic. In other words, because the analyst is a true believer, he is blind to the persuasive potential of his theoretical beliefs. As a result, group members are reduced to guessing at his "religion" from hints in his comments—an extremely inefficient way of communicating values by which to live.

Unlike members of Synanon or Alcoholics Anonymous, patients in group therapy do not have any special commitment to one another. They do not share a common problem (like drug addiction or alcoholism) and do not face the same catastrophic destiny if they fail. Often, the difficulties in everyday life for which they are seeking help are not dealt with in the group; and there is no help, support, or

[6] I have generally labeled the group leader as a therapist to emphasize that it is his beliefs, rather than any consensus among the members, which make up the group's "religion."

118

stern watchfulness from other members when they get in trouble outside the group. Whatever influence the group does have on its members stems mainly from the relationships which the members develop with one another over the course of many meetings. That is, as the other members of the group become increasingly important to him, a given member has to pay increasing attention to their comments about him. Nevertheless, because the ideology of the group is vague and because the various members have different goals and limited extragroup influence on one another, most group therapy does not offer a potent setting for personal change.

Fortunately, group therapy does have the potential for greatly expanded effectiveness. If the beliefs offered by therapy groups were clearly spelled out and attractive to their members, if the members were working together toward common goals, and if the members could have extragroup contact when difficulties related to the goals arose, the chance of major changes taking place would be much greater. The realization of this potential is illustrated by women's consciousness-raising groups, which are also open-ended, limited contact groups, but whose structure more closely approximates the ideal just described.

The goal of women's consciousness-raising groups is to increase their members' understanding of women's oppression. Because all the members are women, they share a variety of problems; and because a group's goal is explicit, the members have by joining indicated a shared commitment to it. Although consciousness-raising groups vary widely, in their approach to the goal most groups deal with two main areas. The relative emphasis given to each varies, but most such groups conduct both an intimate discussion of the personal problems of their members—as these relate to problems of women in general—and a more abstract discussion of women's role in the larger political context. Contacts between members outside the group are not discouraged; and I am told by a friend with extensive experience in

119

women's groups that such contacts are common in the more successful ones.

The goal of women's consciousness-raising groups has nothing to do with therapy for their members. In fact, many leaders of the women's movement would insist that little can be done to help individual women until the inequities affecting all women are corrected. Nevertheless, many women have achieved new self-confidence and greater effectiveness in their work and home lives as a result of participating in such groups. I believe that such results are not accidental but are the consequence of a group structure well designed for changing the beliefs and behavior of its members (that is, given the structure of the groups, the discussion of personal problems is likely to lead to constructive suggestions for change, group pressures toward implementing the change, and group support in maintaining the change). If therapy groups were to undergo parallel changes in their structure, I would expect them to have a correspondingly greater impact on their members' lives.

The recent spate of marathons, T-groups, and human relations workshops has called attention to *fixed duration, limited contact groups*. They resemble open-ended, limited contact groups except that they meet only once or at most for a prearranged, small number of times.

Despite the perplexing variety of these groups, it is fair to say that their rapid spread, which has been characterized by an emphasis on "touchie-feelie" techniques, has taken on the proportions of a new religious movement, a kind of secular revivalism. Its dogma requires believers to place great value on their sensory experiences and, in interactions with others, on personal authenticity and intimacy of contact. As the movement has spread, its evangelists have increasingly advocated the creation of a new subculture to foster such values. Clearly, the "group grope" groundswell is a protest against the computerized alienation of contemporary life. Nevertheless, though I sympathize with these

120

values, the attempt to implement them by a religious movement seems to me to be doomed to failure in a manner similar to the withering of the flower children in the late 1960s. A more reasonable approach would appear to be political action aimed at achieving the sorts of social changes that would allow such values to flourish.

Fixed duration, limited contact groups do, however, have their own combination of advantages and disadvantages. These groups offer for a fee a special setting in which members can experience a few hours of the excitement of intense human contact. This emotional experience is restricted to a specific time and place and precludes the possibility of long-term participation. In this sense, paying for the excitement of such an experience is no different from paying for the excitement of experiencing a roller coaster ride, a sexy movie, or a double martini. As long as the group members realize that they are paying for fun instead of personal change, such groups provide a welcome respite from the bureaucratic inhumanities of contemporary life.

As far as actual therapeutic benefits are concerned, the fixed duration of such groups may for some people increase the pressure toward change. That is, if they enter a group expecting help with their problems, the time limitation may lead them to discuss sensitive material more rapidly, listen to the group's suggestions more attentively, and experiment with new ways of behaving more readily than would otherwise be the case. In this manner, a process of personal change might be set in motion which would continue after the group dissolved. The likelihood of such change actually occurring of course increases if the group's goals are both modest and explicit (for example, overcoming anxiety about speaking in public).

When the goals are vague, the promise of a quick cure, implied by the group's brief duration, can give its members unrealistically high expectations of change. In this way, credulous members may be set up for a severe dis-

121

appointment when the group dissolves and their hopes remain unfulfilled. Certainly, any person who concludes, "I guess I must be a hopeless case," has not been helped by his experience. Because the goals of fixed duration, limited contact groups are typically vague (for example, fulfilling human potentiality or expanding self-awareness) and because the members have no commitment to one another beyond the brief time duration of the group, such groups probably engender little or no long-term improvements in their members beyond those fortuitously set into motion by the placebo effect.

Group Process. The term *group process* is used to denote the kinds of interactions that take place within a given group—that is, the form rather than the content of the group's interactions. There are two types of interaction: between the leader and the rest of the group and among the various group members. In the first, the leader may influence the beliefs and behavior of group members by giving expert advice or information, by encouraging or discouraging specific kinds of interactions among group members, by initiating group healing rituals, or by any of a variety of other means. He may even use the ploy of passivity (for example, insisting that he is just another member of the group or that he is merely a consultant, not a leader) as a means of compelling group members to deal explicitly with the problem of leadership while enhancing his aura of mystery by making so perplexing a pronouncement. Similarly, group members may offer suggestions to one another, attack one another verbally, give testimonials, express feelings, participate in group healing rituals, or interact in a variety of other ways, including getting in touch with one another outside the group.

The precise nature of the process within any particular group is determined by a number of broad factors above and beyond personality variations among its members. For example, the group's structure is of great importance in determining the kinds of interactions which take place among members. Thus, although extragroup contact has no place in fixed duration, limited contact groups, it forms the core of what goes on in a total environment. Similarly, the leader's beliefs (for example, it is good to express emotions) lead him to influence group process by encouraging certain types of interactions while discouraging others.

Surprisingly, however, many a group leader sees himself as the captain of a rudderless ship afloat on an uncharted ocean. Although this view, which is expressed in such terms as "I just respond to the here and now," certainly makes each group into an adventure, it also increases the likelihood of the group's going nowhere or of foundering on unexpected shoals. I believe that this view of group process as essentially unpredictable and out of the leader's control is an accurate one for the great majority of groups because their goals are vague or unspecified.

The goal of a typical group might be something like helping members to become better adjusted. Because such an aim is devoid of content, neither the leader nor the group members have any way of knowing whether what they are doing at a given moment is getting them any closer to better adjustment. In this situation, the leader's strategy is a simple one: He waits expectantly (or wearily) for something to develop to which he can respond. Meanwhile, group members wait tensely, uncertain about what is expected of them. Finally, someone says something—almost anything will do— and when another member responds, the group is underway. Gradually more and more people join in—agreeing, disagreeing, changing the subject, and commenting on one another—while everyone periodically eyes the leader to check on his approval. Eventually the leader comments on what has taken place, and then his comment becomes the topic of further discussion. In this way, the group fills up its allotted time, with occasional moments of emotional drama punctuating the activities. No wonder the leaders of such groups view group process as unpredictable. Because the members do not know what to do, they begin trial-and-error experimentation to see what the leader expects from them. But because he has no expectations, the group continues to drift on like a rudderless ship.

It may be argued that, because the leader has no expectations, the members' "neurotic" behavior will fail to gain his approval—leading them to try out new and "healthier" ways of interacting. Of course, the members might equally well try out even more "neurotic" ways of interacting; and even if they acted "healthier," a leader without any expectations would ignore their improved behavior too. Furthermore, even if the members did try acting "healthier" in relation to one another and even if the leader did approve of such interactions, there is no reason that the members should then act "healthier" outside the group, where they are beset by real problems in a setting quite different from that of the group.

Similarly, it might be argued that the patterns of interaction within the group will mirror the kinds of problems the members have outside the group. Such a parallel does not always occur, but, even when it does, it will not necessarily lead to "better adjustment" of the participants. Rather, any pattern of interaction that is repeated in session after session suggests that the participants have found a way of filling time that is acceptable to the leader. Persons uninitiated into the paradoxical mysteries of therapy may have difficulty in believing the incredible stretches of time that therapists can wait "for the resistance to end" while their individual patients or groups plod on in the same rut, doggedly believing that they are doing the right thing.

The problem of the unpredictability of group process disappears when a group has concrete goals. Consider, for example, a group whose goal is overcoming anxiety about public speaking. In a group such as this, where the members share a particular problem, there is a sense of common motivation which is absent from most groups. At different times, the group process might involve a discussion of the sources of anxiety in public speaking, individual practice in giving talks before the rest of the group followed by specific comments from group members on the strong and weak points of each presentation, a critical discussion of readings on public speaking, systematic desensitization of a group hierarchy of members' fears, or a variety of similar, goal-related activities. In such a group, both the leader and the members understand what they are doing and why they are doing it. Although digressions may be accepted for a few minutes because they may lead to something of use to the group as a whole, once they turn out to be unproductive, the group leader can tactfully shift the direction of the group back to goal-related activities. Furthermore, the clear relationship of the group's activities to its stated goals enhances the placebo value of those activities. That is, even if some of the activities have no intrinsic validity in reducing anxiety about public speaking, their reassuring appearance of validity may calm the members sufficiently for them briefly to be successful in public speaking; and the increased confidence resulting from such successes may in turn lead to a more permanent diminution of anxiety.

In short, then, of all the factors affecting group process, group goals seem to me to be both the most important and the most neglected. Consequently, if groups formed around more concretely specified goals, I would expect group process to become both less chaotic and more functional: there's smooth sailing ahead when the ship hits the plan.

Individual Faith-Healing versus Group Faith-Healing. Because the first seven chapters of this book are concerned with individual therapy, I am including this brief summary in the hope that it will offer a useful comparison of placebo therapy in individual and group settings.

In individual therapy, the goals are agreed upon

separately with each patient, and placebo communications are tailored to his personal beliefs. In the group setting, goals are set for the group as a whole, and the persuasive power of communication is based on the group's ideology. Hopefully, both the group's goals and its ideology are sufficiently explicit so that only people who wish to attain its goals and who believe in its ideology become members. Thus, instead of fitting the placebo communication to the patient, the patients are selected to fit the placebo communication. Still, there is great individual variation among people with ostensibly similar problems. For example, one person may fear speaking in public because he is afraid of being laughed at, while someone else may have the same fear because he does not know how to go about organizing a speech. Similarly, there is great variation among people who are sympathetic to a given set of beliefs, as is illustrated by the differences in religious beliefs among the members of any congregation. Therefore, because of the specificity that exists in the one-to-one setting, placebo communications in individual therapy are more precise, and consequently more effective, than in groups. A similar argument points to the greater precision and effectiveness of healing rituals in the one-to-one setting.

In individual therapy, only the therapist is a source of pressure toward and support for change, while in groups the other members add their own multifaceted pressure and support. Furthermore, when the entire group shares similar problems, goals, and beliefs, other members become an important reference group for each individual. Thus, although both the individual therapist and the group leader work for change from an exalted, one-up position, the pressure toward and support for change which comes from a peer group is a resource uniquely available to the group therapist.

Finally, individual therapy involves a relatively small intrusion into the patient's moment-to-moment existence, but groups vary in their degree of intrusion according to their structure. At one extreme, the total environment affects virtually every aspect of its members' lives, while at the other extreme, fixed duration, limited contact groups have a minimal impact. Thus, the range of influence offered by different groups is broader than that offered by different types of individual therapy.

In summary, while opportunities for faith-healing abound in both individual and group settings, differences between the settings point to somewhat different placebo strategies as most effective in each context.

NINE

Applications to
Mass Audiences

As members of a common culture, we share many beliefs which are so obvious as to remain unnoticed in everyday life. When these beliefs are challenged, they are defended as self-evident. For example, Americans are revolted at the thought of eating bats despite their nutritional advantages, while members of bat-eating cultures are similarly sickened in disbelief at some of our culinary delights. These pervasive beliefs, of which food preferences are only one example, can be characterized in the terms of this book as our common faith.

I have argued that therapeutic communications based on people's faith lead to changes in their beliefs and behavior. In everyday life, the communications of the mass media continually change beliefs and behavior in our mass culture. Political polls, for example, record the weekly changes in the beliefs of millions of people, and on election day these beliefs are transformed into the symbolic behavior of lever-pulling. A less awesome example of the effect of such mass communications can be seen in the recent widespread use of genital deodorants. In this case, Americans' obsession with bodily functioning, odors, and dirt has been cunningly used in a mass antipublic—and antipubic—health campaign which has led to an increase in numerous gynecological maladies. Although these beliefs have been similarly exploited to sell a myriad of dubious pills and emollients, and may even be a factor in the spread of drug abuse, the beliefs probably have also helped stimulate public responsiveness to warnings about the dangers of pollution.

Among the many topics about which millions of people receive mass communications is mental health. These communications are conveyed through television and radio programs as well as columns and articles in newspapers and magazines while numerous educational, charitable, and religious organizations spread their messages on mental health in meetings and publications. One can hardly avoid the advice on how to handle life's problems which constantly streams in from psychologists, psychiatrists, religious leaders, and astrologers. Because this deluge shows no sign of abating, it is interesting to speculate about the possibility of using the principles of placebo therapy to divert some of that flood into more productive channels (although my experience with mass communications is almost exclusively that of a recipient, the potential implications of placebo principles in this area are sufficiently important for me to acquiesce to the temptation to write about them).

The uses of mass placebo communications depend on the kinds of audiences which receive them. Mass audiences differ from groups in that the direction of communication is almost exclusively from the speaker[1] to the audience, and physical circumstances make impossible a dialogue either between him and each individual in the audience or between every possible pair of audience members. Given that communications flow in one direction, from the speaker to the audience, the audiences can be divided into two types. The first, mass meetings, consists of those audiences who are assembled in a particular place at a particular time around a common point of attention; the second type of audience consists of those individuals who are exposed to a given communication in the mass media, albeit at widely disparate times and places.

Because all the people at a mass meeting are gathered together at a particular place and time, such meetings bear at least some resemblance to the groups already discussed. People usually attend meetings because they are sympathetic to, or at least interested in, the point of view to be expressed. Thus, audiences are self-selecting for receptivity to a speaker's message in a manner similar to the self-selection of groups. Furthermore, people who come to a meeting display by their attendance—and sometimes even payment of money —some degree of involvement in what takes place. Naturally, the involvement may be rather slight because the secure anonymity of an audience demands less from its members than does the personal scrutiny of a group, but even this involvement is sufficient to enhance an audience's already heightened receptivity to the speaker's message. Finally, although the members of an audience do not speak to one another on any mass basis, the many visible and audible signs of an audience's mood constitute a potent force at any meet-

[1] I am using the term *speaker* to designate the source of mass communications even though the source may be a group of people or a wordless picture, just as I have used *leader* for groups and *therapist* for one-to-one interactions. Although the appropriateness of such labels varies with the context in which they are used, it is convenient for the sake of discussion to have consistent terminology available.

ing. This mood, which may rise to fervent and even frenzied proportions at political and religious meetings, acts on each individual in a manner similar to the way group pressures function in a group setting: Believers are spurred on even further, those wavering may be swept along with the rest of the crowd, and doubters, if not persuaded, are at least silenced.

Despite these parallels between mass meetings and groups, the effect of a speaker's placebo communications on his audience must obviously be even weaker than that of a leader's placebo communications on group members. Although a group leader has difficulty in formulating a placebo communication for the group as a whole because the beliefs of the various members are not identical, he has at least had some face-to-face contact with each of them. In this way, his knowledge of their beliefs enables him to formulate the best group communication possible under the circumstances. A speaker, however, rarely knows more than a few of the members of his audience. For this reason, his persuasive communications can be based only on the most general and widely held beliefs and on the limited information provided by the audience's mood (though even when an audience is "with" a speaker, he may not know what he is doing right).

Such a speaker who attempts to improve the mental health of his audience by communications based on cultural generalities is a far cry from a therapist who is trying to help one patient with specific problems by communications based on the patient's unique beliefs. Thus, because a mass meeting is neither individual nor group therapy, the speaker's effectiveness must be judged by a different and more appropriate standard.

In measuring the effectiveness of individual or group therapy, it is important to remember that all patients have come for help with their problems. Therefore, the effect of therapy on all patients must be averaged together and com-

131

pared with the effect of some other treatment—or no treatment at all—on another group of people with comparable problems. In contrast, many people attending a meeting concerned with mental health do not have problems with which they want help, so averaging the speaker's effect on the audience would be inappropriate. A more reasonable way of assessing the speaker's effect would be to see how many members of the audience benefited from his talk and how great their benefit was. If he helped more people at a cost of less money and professional time per person than would be possible by other modes of treatment, he would have to be judged effective. His degree of effectiveness, in turn, would be measured by the extent of savings in money and professional time per person helped.

A lecture that I gave a few years ago as part of an introductory psychology course should help to illustrate these ideas. As is unfortunately the case in an increasing number of undergraduate courses in this country, my class was composed of over six hundred students. We met in a huge lecture hall, with both orchestra and balcony sections, and I spoke with a microphone from an elevated stage.

The lecture was devoted to the therapeutic uses of relaxation-training and systematic desensitization. Although the lecture was factual in content, it was organized in a persuasive manner; that is, my goal was not merely to convey current knowledge about the techniques but also to persuade my students that they were good. During the last part of the period, I demonstrated a relaxation induction with the entire class.[2] As I suggested that the students relax various parts of their bodies, the background murmur rapidly disappeared, and the lecture hall became amazingly silent.

After the demonstration was over, the students left

---

[2] Naturally, I told the students that participation was voluntary and that those who did not wish to take part could either leave first or sit quietly and observe. No one left, and only a handful of the students kept their eyes open.

the hall quietly—in marked contrast to their usual uproar. Several students came up to the stage to tell me that relaxation is "great stuff." Although I had hoped that some of the more anxious students might practice relaxation on their own, I made no such suggestion during my lecture because I felt that it would be out of place in the context of an academic course. The farthest that I felt I could legitimately go was to try to persuade the students by both facts and their own personal experience that some of the newer approaches to therapy are worthwhile even though they violate current therapeutic stereotypes.

Despite my hesitation, evidence of the positive effects of the demonstration began to mount. Over a period of time, a number of students sought me out to tell me of their experiences with relaxation. One student, for example, told me that he had had a test in the class that followed my lecture. He said that he usually did not do well on tests, despite studying carefully, because he became very anxious during exams. He explained that his anxiety made it hard for him to concentrate and that he was unable to remember material he could recall after the test when he was more relaxed. As a result of the relaxation demonstration, however, he had taken his test while still feeling calm. He reported happily that he had gotten an "A" on the exam and that he had subsequently relaxed before other exams to good effect. A number of students described similar positive experiences and said that they had been practicing the relaxation exercise ever since the lecture. In fact, when I ran a demonstration group at one of the university dormitories a year later, a student from that lecture joined the group and brought his roommate with him. He told me that he had been practicing relaxing ever since my lecture and that he had used relaxation to overcome anxiety in a number of academic and interpersonal areas. He had also taught his roommate how to relax, and the roommate was now relaxing before tests.

Despite the fragmentary nature of these reports—I

know nothing about the reactions of 98 percent of the students—the results are encouraging. Because I was paid by the university anyway and would have given the lecture even if it had improved no one's mental health, any good effects were gravy and were achieved at the expense of no money or professional time whatsoever (lectures do not generally help people with their problems, and the students' unusual reaction to the demonstration suggests that my lectures are typically just as unhelpful as those of my colleagues).

The apparent success of this lecture suggests that a speaker can make use of the therapeutic opportunities present in mass meetings. His strategy would be to devote part of his talk to teaching the audience how to perform a healing ritual for a common type of problem. Because the ritual is for a common problem, any mass meeting will contain some people who should profit from it. Naturally, the larger the meeting, the greater the number of people helped.

The idea of presenting placebo communications and healing rituals to mass meetings has obvious implications for the mass media. However, for many reasons the impact of placebo communications is more diluted in the mass media than in any of the other settings thus far discussed. First, there is less control over the recipients of such communications than at mass meetings. People who watch a given TV program or read a particular newspaper are much more varied than the audience at a particular meeting; communications in the mass media reach people from different subcultures, who differ from one another in a number of important beliefs. Because the effectiveness of placebo communications depends on their being grounded in their recipients' beliefs, certain segments of the audience will not be persuaded by what they hear. In fact, a boomerang effect can be predicted for the subgroups who hold beliefs opposite to those on which the communications are based.

Moreover, listening to the radio or reading a magazine requires even less personal involvement than does attending a meeting. People's casual, almost absent-minded relationship to the mass media—radio and TV function largely as background noise for many families—diminishes the impact of communications from these sources. And, because the audience for a given mass communication is not assembled at a particular place and time, there is no audience mood for the individual to feel and be swayed by. This lack further diminishes the impact of communications in the mass media.

One last element, which is present in all settings but which predominates in the mass media, further weakens the persuasive effect of mass communications. That element is the high frequency with which people avoid messages that they find boring or unpleasant. Newspaper readers skip over articles and advertisements; TV viewers switch channels, drink beer, and converse. This distractibility is minimized in interpersonal settings by situational pressures. Thus, in a one-to-one conversation, the social pressures to listen to the other person are intense. Inattenation is a serious faux pas and obliges the transgressor not only to prolong by apologies the discussion he wishes to escape but also to listen with concerned attention to a repetition of the remarks he has ignored. Similarly, group pressures also function to maintain members' alert involvement, and the dominant position which a speaker occupies at a mass meeting ensures that at least an important part of his message is heard by those in the audience. Only the somnolent are insulated from his words; and audience pressures are such that even the most narcogenic speaker renders insensible a mere scattering of his listeners. In contrast, newspapers and television sets are inanimate and do not protest when their pages are turned or their channels switched. In the absence of countervailing situational pressures, distractibility and selective inattention thrive among mass media audiences and further diminish the impact of mass communications.

To say that the effect of messages in the media on the

individual is less than that in any other setting is not to say that is is nonexistent. For example, even among mass media audiences there is some self-selection; the act of watching a program or buying a magazine entails a slight degree of involvement and commitment. Furthermore, the inattention of mass media audiences to unpleasant communications paradoxically implies that any members who do actually attend to a given message are likely to be influenced by it. These elements of self-selection ensure that mass media audiences have beliefs that are more receptive to the messages before them than equally large audiences chosen at random.

Although there is no audience mood to sway the individual, similar, though weaker forces are at work in the mass media. Television, for example, often records shows before live audiences, so that the sounds of laughter or brief pictures of rapt attention can influence the solitary viewer. More importantly, evidence from studies of the mass media suggests that the impact of communications takes place in a two-step fashion. Opinion leaders in the community are influenced directly by the mass media, while others are affected by personal contact with the opinion leaders. In other words, the influence of a particular communication does not end with those who are directly exposed to it; in the process of word-of-mouth transmission, potent interpersonal forces are enlisted to magnify its impact.

Finally, mass media audiences are so much larger than any others discussed, frequently running into the tens of millions, that the slightest impact of a particular massage is of tremendous importance. If a particular psychological technique or placebo communication helped even 1 percent of a given audience, many thousands would benefit; and that number might well be increased as opinion leaders spread the good word.

Drama, news, and advice-giving are the main formats in which personal problems are treated (in both senses of the word) by the mass media. The following brief discussion looks at each of these areas with placebo principles in mind.

Soap operas and other dramatic offerings on radio and television, as well as magazine fiction and newspaper cartoons, all deal directly with people's problems and the attempts of experts to help them. Laboratory experimentation has demonstrated that similar dramatic presentations have a considerable effect on the subsequent behavior of audience members[3], so it is reasonable to assume that such effects also exist in the mass media. A recent unsystematic and boring examination of some of these dramas has suggested to me, however, that what they offer—and hence what audiences can learn from them—is not especially helpful.

These mass dramatic events provide a demonstration of role relationships in therapy. They show how to talk about personal problems and how the quiet but omniscient therapist can magically help people in distress. Although the stereotypes presented are often overly specific, inaccurate, or misleading, even the most accurate portrayal would be of little use because such displays about therapy function as professional advertisements rather than as potential resources for people with problems. In this way the dramatizations are no different from similar flattering ones of the work of lawyers, physicians, and policemen.

Practically the only suggestion for action implicit in such dramatizations is "if you have a problem, see a therapist." This suggestion, which encourages an attitude of helplessness toward one's own problems, may not be especially harmful to those few in the audience who do see therapists, but it is certainly unfortunate for those who lead lives of

---

[3] This kind of learning, referred to as *observational learning* or *modeling,* has been shown to have rapid effects on both the acquisition and performance of a wide variety of behavior. In addition, modeling has already proven therapeutically effective in such diverse areas as reducing adults' fears and teaching language to nonverbal autistic children. Some references about modeling are included in the Annotated Bibliography.

quiet desperation. Furthermore, the notion that only an expert can be of help with personal problems is usually linked to the suggestion that hangups are so awesome or ineffable that they constitute a treasured badge of uniqueness. In my work with college students, for example, I frequently encountered the following chain of reasoning: Some geniuses are hungup weirdos. [True.] For me to be worthwhile, I have to be a genius. [Nonsense.] I have some hangups which make me miserable. [True.] If I get rid of these hangups, I will no longer be miserable. [Probably true.] But by losing these hangups I will lose my unique genius. [Both illogical and nonsensical.] Therefore, I must be either a hungup, miserable, worthwhile genius or a worthless, contented cow. [This is the sort of conclusion one reaches after an illogical and unscrutinized chain of thoughts.] Oh, the agony of being faced with such a choice! [After generating such drivel, it is fun to slobber in it.] By perpetuating a similar linkage between personal misery and individuality, creativity, genius, or other laudable characteristics, the dramatic clichés of the mass media do a disservice to their audiences.

Mass dramatizations could foster more constructive beliefs and behavior in a number of ways. Essentially, such improvements involve demonstrating in action the therapeutic principles thus far discussed. For example, portrayals of therapy could show the therapist teaching his patients to observe their own behavior. When the woman in the soap opera says, "I just can't cope with life, Doctor," the therapist does not have to reply, "How does it feel to be unable to cope?" He could instead say, "Tell me about a recent situation that you were unable to cope with." Then, when the woman describes a visit from her mother-in-law, the therapist could have her focus on the minutiae of who said what to whom and what happened next. Gradually, the woman could come to see more clearly the intricacies of the situation and discuss more effective ways of handling some of her mother-in-law's most devastating ploys. Surely, such a treatment lends itself to flashbacks and other dramatic techniques as smoothly as the "how does X feel?" response. And in the repeated process of watching people learn to observe behavior and benefit from their observations, members of the audience might well learn to do the same.

Another useful addition would be to have audiences observe the therapist and patient engage in problem-solving discussions aimed at developing coping strategies. When the suburban housewife declares to her therapist (and her TV audience of other suburban housewives) that she is desperately lonely at home while the children are at school and her husband is at work, the therapist need not search for a clue in her distant past. Instead, he could initiate a discussion aimed at discovering ways of meaningfully using her time and meeting other people (the difficulty of solving such a problem is considerable and is probably an important determinant of "sin in the suburbs"). Hopefully, discussions such as these would lead some audience members to consider tackling their own problems in a similar, constructive way.

Finally, such dramatic settings offer an ideal opportunity for the mass demonstration of simple healing rituals. Thus, the therapist could tell his anxious patient, "I'm going to show you how to relax. Once you've learned this exercise, you can use it to calm yourself whenever you get tense." As he teaches his patient how to relax on TV, some anxious members of the audience might decide to try the exercise themselves.

Mental health issues are frequently presented as news in the mass media. Television and radio newscasts and articles in newspapers and news magazines all catalog the latest Kafkaesque horrors in state mental hospitals or the debut of new therapeutic drugs and techniques. Special, longer programs in the electronic media and articles of general interest in numerous periodicals also provide the public with mental health information. Finally, public service advertisements in all of the mass media proclaim helpful

139

slogans, such as "alcoholism is a disease; cover your mouth and you won't catch it."

Information coming from these sources differs in two important ways from that conveyed by drama. The first is that the information is more credible to its audiences. Because news is supposed to be factual and because it comes from real psychologists and psychiatrists (as opposed to actors playing the roles of experts), audiences are much more likely to believe what they see and hear. In the field of medicine, for example, the recent vitamin C fad was begun by news publicity, not by use of the vitamin in TV hospital dramas. The second difference is that, in the area of personal problems, news sources tend to convey only abstract information with no discernible implications for action. In effectual as mental health dramas may be, they at least show prospective therapeutic patients how to enter an office gloomily, stare sadly at the floor while telling their story, and not peek at the therapist's face to see his reaction. News presentations tend to be more of the form "at an international mental health forum yesterday, Dr. X presented a new therapeutic technique for the treatment of depression. Seven smiling ex-patients expressed their enthusiasm for this new treatment." Unfortunately, such reports give no clue to the many sad people in the audience as to what to do to become as happy as those treated by Dr. X. Similarly, although public service advertisements concerning mental health originate from highly credible public or charitable organizations, they rarely contain useful information for the suffering members of their audience (some advertisements do encourage improved conditions for people with severe problems—for example, "hire former mental patients"—but this indirect benefit does not compensate for the lack of communications aimed directly at them).

Unfortunately, the high credibility characterizing these sources of information is wasted because of the abstract nature of the messages conveyed. The discussions of placebo principles presented in this book do, however, suggest how to make therapeutic use of this credibility: by demonstrating healing rituals. Because the source of the rituals is credible, those in the audience who try them will have faith that they will work. And this faith in turn makes it more likely that people will actually benefit.

This goal can best be accomplished in news stories by including sufficient information for readers to try the healing ritual. Thus, a newspaper article might include: "Dr. Y was successful in helping stutterers by having them practice speaking slowly to the regular beat of a metronome—for example, 'Four score and se-ven years ago. . . .' Once they were able to speak in this way without stuttering, they gradually practiced increasing the speed of their speech and making the rhythm ever closer to that of English."

Television newscasts and special programs could add greatly to the impact of such healing rituals by showing them in use with appropriate patients. In doing so, they could use the persuasive power of films which illustrate the effects of the technique under consideration. Thus, it would be easy to make a brief five-part film showing a stutterer's speech before he learned the technique, Dr. Y teaching him to use the metronome, his speech after a week's practice, his normal speech after several weeks, and his normal speech a year after having used the technique. Finally, interviews with experts, which form the basis of so much news, could be conducted so as to include enough of the details of healing rituals for audience members to try them. All too often, a technique is sketchily presented, and the bulk of the discussion is devoted to how the technique was discovered, research on its effectiveness, and other abstract considerations.

The advice-giving format has always been a popular one in the mass media and has generally dealt with personal problems. Advice has been offered by mental health experts, religious leaders, and other well-meaning and not-so-well-

141

meaning people. The marketability of newspaper and magazine columns as well as the weekday glut of advice-giving programs on radio and TV attest to the public appetite for such fare.

Advice-giving in the mass media differs from drama and news in a number of respects. Perhaps the most important of these is that part of its format is an explicit interaction between the advice giver and specific, albeit faceless, members of the audience. This aspect of the advice-giving format retains its importance even when it is phony (for example, when the "lady from Nebraska who writes to ask about her husband's roving eye" is really a man from New Jersey in the advice giver's employ). The point of responding to particular audience members is to encourage the rest of the audience to view the advice as directed toward their peers, who may at that moment be reading the same column or watching the same television program. In fact, individuals in the audience frequently have fantasies about the person being advised ("I hope he's listening now") or about the advice giver ("I like her in general, but she doesn't seem to understand how a mother-in-law feels"). In this way, faithful members of the audience build up over time individual images of the advice giver and gradually develop a sense of trust in his judgment.

This sense of trust makes information obtained from an advice-giving format more credible than that from dramatic settings. Of course, since advice consists of what one ought to do, while news supposedly is made up of facts, news sources still remain the most credible of the three. This hierarchy of credibility is an interesting feature of contemporary mass culture. I would guess that it is the result of the high value we place on facts even if they may turn out to be wrong, misleading, or meaningless. Perhaps this emphasis reflects the scientistic faith of our electronic age.

Unlike the other mass media sources, advice-giving

by definition involves concrete suggestions for action. This feature is more complex than it at first appears. Surely, the advice is not given primarily for the benefit of the person seeking it; in some cases, no such person even exists. And when someone does write to ask for help, putting the advice in a syndicated column is certainly an odd way of lending a hand. Obviously, the real function of the advice is to provide entertainment for those in the audience not seeking help rather than guidance for those who do seek it. In this way, advice-giving can be seen as comparable to drama, while the feelings of the audience about the advice giver and the advisee resemble those about characters in a play.

The advice-giving format does, however, have great potential for helping members of mass audiences with their problems. Here is a setting devoted to personal problems where the words of the advice giver are reasonably well trusted and where the advice is directed to the audience as a whole. The only change of emphasis needed is from gearing the advice solely to the audience's entertainment to both entertainment and possible benefit (as long as the possibility of benefit is provided for, the size of the audience virtually guarantees that some people will be helped).

Enabling some people to benefit could be accomplished in a number of ways, all of which involve altering the advice-giving format in accord with the new emphasis in its goals. First, both the problems dealt with and the advice offered are usually too specific to be relevant to many people. A suggestion such as "I'm afraid you'll have to invite your aunt to the party this time" may charm the audience by its wisdom but is unlikely to enlighten many of them because few people have similar problems with their aunts in similar situations. Furthermore, the intricacies of a particular person's specific problem are usually too subtle, multifarious, or exotic to be conveyed in a letter to an advice giver. Thus, when the problems discussed are those of real people, offer-

143

ing such specific solutions can be irresponsible because a particular detail omitted from the letter may invalidate the recommended course of action.

In contrast, an approach of discussing general types of problems and offering general strategies for solving them avoids these objections. For example, an advice giver on television might announce, "A number of viewers have written to ask what they can do about the fears they have. They have complained of fear of heights, of crowds, of riding in airplances or cars, of animals, and of numerous other things that upset them. Such fears are quite common, and, though they may be unpleasant, they are nothing to worry about. Fortunately, a number of techniques exist which have enabled many people to rid themselves of the annoyance of such fears." He could then go on to explain systematic desensitization and tell people how to go about desensitizing their own fears. This approach once again illustrates an important advantage of healing rituals: the self-direction of change. Instead of the advice giver's conveying specific instructions (which might be offbase, confirming the individual's belief that he cannot help himself), he can offer a general strategy of self-help and allow each individual to adapt it to his own needs.

Another area in which change would be desirable, primarily on television shows, is the excessively verbal emphasis of the advice-giving format. As already mentioned, demonstrations of healing rituals are more effective than verbal descriptions of them. There is no reason that either the advice giver or an actor could not show what a particular healing ritual looks like once it has been described. In fact, the uninterrupted display of the advice giver's talking face is an unimaginative use of a primarily visual medium, so this kind of alteration in the format would increase its entertainment value while making it possible for audience members to benefit.

Finally, although some healing rituals appear to be

144

valid apart from any placebo enhancement, others may depend entirely on placebo principles for their effectiveness. In the case of the latter, the advice giver would have to show considerable ingenuity in devising new and different techniques because, as the audience grew familiar with a given ritual, its effectiveness would diminish. (An individual therapist can use an old technique with a new patient because it is new to him, but this novelty is lost after it is presented to a mass audience.) Of course, audiences do change over time, and, after a number of years, a forgotten healing ritual can be resurrected. For example, in the 1920s a hypnotist named Emile Coué devised the "universal suggestion": Every day, in every way, I'm getting better and better. His healing ritual, which swept Europe and America at the time, consisted of saying the suggestion to oneself over and over several times a day. Each person was to understand the suggestion as having special relevance to his own personal problems. Thus, a man with headaches knew that he was practicing the suggestion to get rid of his headaches (although he was aware that he might derive other, perhaps unexpected, benefits from it); a shy woman knew that she was primarily practicing to become more socially confident.

Because today's college students were born after Coué had been forgotten and because many of them are fascinated by meditation, I decided to try the universal suggestion again. I spoke to the demonstration group mentioned earlier about meditation, chanting, altered states of consciousness, and hypnosis. After indicating similarities and differences among them, I pointed out that, by chanting the universal suggestion, one could derive both the contemplative advantages of meditation and the suggestive advantages of self-hypnosis. At the follow-up meeting a week later, a young man who had looked rather glum the first time said that he had tried the meditation exercise and that it had relieved his depression. When he did the exercise, however, he felt as if he were just cheering himself up. I smiled and responded, "I see. When you tell yourself you're getting better and better, that's just cheering yourself up; but when you tell yourself you're worthless, that's real honesty." He seemed surprised at first but then indicated that he had received my message. Experiences such as this suggest that healing rituals like Coué's could be effective when presented in an advice-giving format (naturally, when the universal suggestion is presented, its implications for ameliorating depression should be pointed out too—as I have done here).

In summary, just as placebo principles can be applied in individual and group therapy, they have applications for mass meetings and the mass media. In each case, the application depends on the characteristics of the patient, group, or audience involved. Because the mass media are a fact of life and do have an effect on people's problems, the effect should be at least partially therapeutic; and several ways were suggested for using placebo principles in achieving this end.

TEN

Ethical Issues

Any discussion of ethical issues in psychotherapy must begin with a consideration of why the mental health professions exist at all. In one sense, the reason is that the state has taken affirmative legal action to permit their existence, regulate their activities, and encourage their growth. This explanation still leaves unanswered the question of why governments should devote their resources to licensing laws, training and research grants, and similar subsidies of education and treatment. The important sociopolitical function which such expenditures are supposed to support would appear to be the control of noncriminal deviance.

In any society, there are bound to be people who, though breaking no laws, are frightening, disgusting, or otherwise obnoxious to their fellow man. Usually, these people are upsetting because they break one or more of society's unwritten rules. Such deviance causes anxiety in others be-

147

cause it challenges their way of life—the only way of life their society offers. For example, the man who tells all who will listen that he is Jesus Christ is an upsetting person. The role he claims as his own is not supposed to be available to mortals in our society, and thus our government has provided the pretext and personnel to cart him away. Freedom of speech may permit him to say what he will; freedom of religion may allow him his beliefs; but, by declaring him sick, society still has a way to isolate him for "treatment." In other words, state mental hospitals serve as nonjails and mental health professionals as nonjailers for the mentally ill noncriminals.

This is not to deny that some people at some times are unable to care for themselves and that society owes them a helping hand. However, hundreds of thousands of men, women, and children are now incarcerated in dungeons that are hospitals in name only. The aid these people receive from the helping professions is in the spirit of "I'd like to help you out; which way did you come in?" or, more precisely, "I'd like to help you out; that's why I'm locking you in."

Many of the people who are currently hospitalized, to their detriment—and at the taxpayer's expense—could function adequately within society. One psychologist used to illustrate this point by describing a woman who successfully avoided hospitalization: One day the police received a telephone call from a frightened woman who asked for someone to come to "get them to stop shooting those rays at me." An officer was dispatched, and, when he arrived, the woman repeated her complaint. "Are you grounded?" the policeman asked her. The woman seemed puzzled and said that she was not. The officer explained that, once she was grounded, the rays could not hurt her. He asked where the rays were coming from, and the woman pointed to a window. He then took some wire he had brought with him, attached it to one side of the window, strung it around the apartment, and attached it to the other side of the window. As he left, he assured her that she was well grounded and that the rays would not bother her anymore. Nothing further was heard from the woman until she called again several years later. She explained that she had recently moved and that they were shooting the rays at her again. She asked whether the police would send over that nice officer to ground her once more. This inspired bit of placebo therapy calmed a frightened woman and saved her from months or years of a far more wretched and degrading existence.

Unfortunately, many policemen would have taken her instead to a state mental hospital, where she would have remained for prolonged "treatment" of her paranoid schizophrenia. Had she been committed, she would have joined other social deviants, most of whom are poor and lack the economic, social, or political resources to care for themselves or to fight commitment proceedings. The hospitals which house such people are usually located in sparsely populated areas, so that, once the human refuse has been swept from the streets of population centers, it can be dumped where it will no longer be an eyesore. In short, we have a social policy of "out of mind, out of sight."

The way our society controls noncriminal deviance is clearly not a laudable one. As a result, the mental health professions have the task of legitimizing their activities as well as fulfilling their parapolice function. One important means for achieving this legitimacy is to use the trappings of professionalism. The strings of diplomas of hospital employees—which represent decades of specialized education—as well as their drugs, electronic equipment, and esoteric jargon serve to disguise the punitive and custodial nature of their institutions. In addition to camouflage, the mental health field uses distraction in legitimizing its main function. It has created a public image of the therapist as a dignified middle class professional in private practice. Most books about therapy—including this one—are primarily concerned with the individual treatment of relatively minor ("neurotic") personal problems. In other words, the problem of major social deviance has been generally neglected, and the neglect has the effect of distracting attention from the plight of state hospital patients. Of course, it is also true that minor deviants threaten to pull less than their full weight in society or even to become major deviants. Thus, by enabling them to continue to function, the mental health professionals do perform a certain service for the state. However, governments are not in the habit of spending huge sums of money just to make people happier; if social deviance were not a problem on a grand scale,[1] the state's investment in coping with it would be vastly diminished.

Because the state allows therapists to exist—and even encourages them to flourish—in order to control deviance, therapy must adjust people to their environment. Any therapy which turned people into revolutionaries would be rapidly condemned, discredited, and outlawed. Although some therapies are said to allow people to become whatever it is within them to be, such assertions are revealed as empty propaganda whenever a patient "discovers" his antisocial nature. Usually, the therapist's ploy is to label such conclusions not as insights but as symptoms (for example, anger compensating for an unconscious feeling of inferiority or Oedipal hostility displaced to present-day authority figures).

The unpleasant fact that society allows therapists to exist in exchange for their adjusting people to society is easy to see throughout the mental health field once one is looking for it. For example, many housewives consult therapists because of desperate feelings of emptiness. Usually, they feel empty because their lives are empty, and they feel desperate

---

[1] It is possible that, as society becomes more complex, fewer people can successfully meet its demands, so that greater numbers break down under the stress. On the other hand, deviance may be more dysfunctional or more noticeable or both in modern urban settings although its incidence has remained unchanged. Whatever the source of the problem, the solution for it has so far been a cruel one.

because they are trapped. When a therapist tells such a woman that she feels empty because of oral deprivation in childhood, he is communicating to her that it is her feelings, not her day-to-day existence, which need changing. Such an interpretation defends the sex roles and family structure which characterize our present society. In this way, the therapist's interpretation has the effect of protecting his license at the expense of his patient's welfare.

The present discussion is not meant to condemn therapists (as opposed to social institutions) for hypocrisy. Most therapists are sincerely motivated by a desire to help their fellow man. However, as members of a culture and a profession, they have many strong beliefs, and this faith enables them to function with little awareness of certain aspects of their work. I have already suggested that true believers make the most effective healers. Thus far, some studies of traditional therapy have yielded disappointing statistics regarding its effectiveness in helping individuals. If healing is viewed as consisting largely of changing beliefs, I would guess that the reason for such results is that the investigators were looking in the wrong place. Research into the effectiveness of therapy in fostering an acceptance of society might well produce more significant findings (there is already some evidence that therapy leads patients to change their values in the direction of their therapists' values).

Despite the cultural predisposition of mental health professionals to conform to the roles assigned them by society, numerous sanctions exist to assure that they do not drift from their course. Although laws governing therapists' activities are extremely important, the sanctions most relevant here are to be found in professional codes of ethics.

Unfortunately, many people think that professional codes of ethics are designed to protect the public. Though they may have that effect in certain cases, it certainly is not their reason for existence. Such codes of ethics are designed to protect the professions from three main dangers. First, and most important, the codes protect the mental health

151

professions from the government. The professions exist to control noncriminal deviance. They are allowed considerable autonomy and status as long as they do their job and refrain from biting the governmental hand that feeds them. If deviants within the professions were allowed to flourish, the government might act against the professions as a whole. Thus, by regulating themselves through formal codes of ethics, the professions are able to escape more punitive governmental regulation. Second, such codes of ethics protect the professions from the self-destruction of internal bickering. Because it is unethical to declare that one is a better therapist than one's colleague or to try to entice a colleague's patients away, therapists are able to live in relative harmony with one another. This result is remarkable inasmuch as the psychotherapy market is every bit as competitive as the automobile market (it might be objected that the mental health professions constitute an oligopoly—but, then, so do automobile manufacturers). Finally, codes of ethics protect the professions—and those professionals who obey them—from the public. As long as a therapist acts ethically, he cannot be sued for being ineffective.

Within the various codes of ethics, principles can be found concerning the therapist's responsibilities to the state, to the profession, and to the individual patient. The considerations of power thus far discussed imply that these principles form a hierarchy. When they conflict, the state comes first, the profession comes next, and the needs of the patient are attended to last.

This unfortunate situation suggests that the ethical ambiguities facing a therapist are at least as great as the substantive ambiguities of his field. Therapists should properly feel ambivalent about their work—though not because it involves faith-healing. Faith-healing exists in all cultures, but therapists dislike thinking of themselves as faith healers primarily because of the low status accorded to that role in our society. While therapists enjoy the high status of scientists and professionals, faith healers suffer a status some-where between that of quacks and that of religious fanatics.[2] The reason that therapists should feel ambivalent about their work is not that they are faith healers, but that they are at least silent partners in a deal which oppresses noncriminal deviants and open participants in the process of adjusting unhappy people to our less-than-perfect society.

Despite social pressures to the contrary, I believe that therapists should work to combat these negative aspects of their role. While recognizing that they are compromised from the start, therapists should, nevertheless, serve as their patients' advocates to society rather than the other way around. Therapists know the conditions in state mental hos-pitals; they should expose rather than defend or apologize for them. They should work for change in those aspects of society which create misery rather than merely helping the miserable to accept their lot. They should fight all forms of institutionalized discrimination—not only that directed against the mentally ill but also racism and other forms of dis-crimination against ethnic minorities, the physically handi-capped, and women. More people have suffered as a result of these and similar social forces than can ever be treated by psy-chotherapy. Therapists who refuse to risk some measure of security by fighting such forces are truly more a part of the problem than a part of the solution.

Every therapist's professional life bears the stamp of his personal hierarchy of values. By putting the welfare of his patients (and potential patients) at the top of his list, a therapist justifies their faith in him. In this way, he is able to feel virtuous about his work, for he is mobilizing his pa-tients' faith for their own personal benefit.

---

[2] Although therapists may not like to think of themselves as faith healers for personal reasons, there are good therapeutic reasons for not ad-vertising themselves as such. By publicly appearing in the higher status role, they can mobilize greater faith in their patients, which can then be used for therapeutic ends.

Annotated Bibliography

Many of the ideas in this book have been expressed elsewhere; what is new is their combination with my own thoughts to form a coherent frame of reference called placebo therapy. Hopefully, this frame of reference will be useful to others in understanding and modifying people's upsetting beliefs and the problems they entail.

For those who are interested in pursing the issues raised by this book in greater detail, I have included this Annotated Bibliography. I have emphasized primarily those books which deal with topics in a broad manner and have omitted entirely references to more microscopically focused research studies. However, several of the books listed are texts which contain extensive bibliographies of experiments for the further study of those readers who are interested in consulting primary sources. I have also included a few nontechnical books for those readers with less background in academic psychology.

I have listed the references by topic in outline form rather than alphabetically in the hope that this arrangement will make it easier to locate an appropriate title. Naturally, my inclusion of a particular book does not imply that I agree with all or even much of the author's conclusions. Rather, I have chosen books relevant to placebo therapy which I found to be intellectually stimulating, or full of useful data, or both.

Clinical Psychology

GENERAL

FRANK, J. D. *Persuasion and Healing: A Comparative Study of Psychotherapy.* (Rev. ed.) Baltimore: Johns Hopkins Press, 1973.

The first edition of this brilliant book, which appeared in 1961, was one of the main starting points for my thinking about placebo therapy. The book describes striking similarities among various forms of psychotherapy, healing in primitive cultures, religious revivalism, thought reform, and the placebo effect.

BERGIN, A. E., AND GARFIELD, S. L. (Eds.) *Handbook of Psychotherapy and Behavior Change: An Empirical Analysis.* New York: Wylie, 1971.

This ambitious volume contains exhaustive reviews of research (through 1970) in virtually every area of psychotherapy. Most of the chapters, including those by the editors, are of extremely high quality, although the chapter on the placebo effect is somewhat limited in its approach. However, the excellent chaper by E. J. Murray and L. I. Jacobson entitled "The Nature of Learning in Traditional and Behavioral Psychotherapy" more than makes up for this defect. Many of the studies cited by Murray and Jacobson lend support to the validity of placebo principles, and, in fact, the authors arrive at similar conclusions. Many other chapters are also relevant to topics I have dealt with (for example, behavior modification, modeling, operant conditioning, and group therapy).

LONDON, P. *The Modes and Morals of Psychotherapy.* New York: Holt, 1964.

This book appears to have foretold the direction in which American psychotherapy would be evolving. The author clearly recognizes the kinds of moral choices faced by psychotherapists and the institution of psychotherapy, and he accurately identifies therapists as constituting a "secular priesthood."

HYPNOSIS

BARBER, T. X. *Hypnosis: A Scientific Approach.* New York: Van Nostrand, 1969.

Through his persistent and incisive experimental work, Theodore Barber has tracked down many of the important antecedent variables which lead to the behavior commonly called hypnotic. In the process of doing so, he has demonstrated that such behavior can be evoked without the use of a hypnotic induction and without the need for the explanatory concept of a trance state. Unfortunately, much of his work has been misunderstood as mere repeated attempts to show that the concept of a trance state is unnecessary. Those interested in placebo therapy, however, would do well to focus their attention on the control groups rather than the experimental groups in his studies. By understanding the kinds of non-hypnotic conditions which enable subjects to engage in unusual "hypnotized" behavior, one gains valuable insight into the ways in which therapists can help their patients make equally dramatic changes.

HALEY, J. (Ed.) *Advanced Techniques of Hypnosis and Therapy: Selected Papers of Milton Erickson, M.D.* New York: Grune and Stratton, 1967.

157

Placebo Therapy

Milton Erickson has become a legendary figure among present-day hypnotists. Although his theoretical conception of hypnosis has not stood up well under recent experimental tests, his clinical inventiveness is an inspiration to all directive psychotherapists. Reading any of his case studies expands one's clinical imagination and helps one to approach afresh patients from whom nothing seems to work.

BEHAVIOR MODIFICATION

ULLMANN, L. P., AND KRASNER, L. *A Psychological Approach to Abnormal Behavior*. Englewood Cliffs, N. J.: Prentice-Hall, 1969.

Part One of this excellent abnormal psychology textbook consists of the best presentation of behavior modification that I have seen. It contains well-reasoned discussions of social learning theory, including a formulation of abnormal behavior, as well as techniques of behavior modification. The chapter most relevant to placebo therapy is entitled "Social Roles and Deviant Behavior: The Role Enactments of Hypnosis, Placebo, Experimenter Bias, and Other Socially Sanctioned 'Abnormal' Behavior."

LAZARUS, A. A. *Behavior Therapy and Beyond*. New York: McGraw-Hill, 1971.

Arnold Lazarus is an admirably pragmatic therapist who gives lucid instruction in applying straightforward techniques to not-so-straightforward cases. His advocacy of "technical eclecticism"—that is, of using any technique that works, even when its theoretical rational is poor—fits in well with placebo therapy. Naturally, I would suggest that many such techniques work because of placebo principles rather than because of any inherent validity in the techniques themselves. Lazarus does advocate maximizing the placebo effect in therapy; and, like Erickson, he has a way with words that allows him to achieve this goal.

BECKER, W. C. *Parents Are Teachers: A Child Management Program*. Champaign, Ill.: Research Press, 1971.

158

Annotated Bibliography

This is a very useful, nontechnical book which explains principles of reinforcement to parents and makes clear and concrete suggestions for handling common problems of childhood.

COMMUNICATIONS THEORY

HALEY, J. *Strategies of Psychotherapy.* New York: Grune and Stratton, 1963.

This rare book is a masterpiece. The author first explains communications theory and then looks at various types of psychotherapy from that vantage point. Jay Haley is both an excellent observer of behavior and an incisive writer with a keen sense of irony. This book should be required reading for all therapists.

WATZLAWICK, P., BEAVIN, J. H., AND JACKSON, D. D. *Pragmatics of Human Communication: A Study of Interactional Patterns, Pathologies, and Paradoxes.* New York: Norton, 1967.

This book contains an excellent formulation of communications theory and many thought-provoking illustrations.

Social Psychology

In discussing placebo therapy, I have made extensive use of the theories, effects, and concepts of social psychology; and I have usually omitted, for stylistic reasons, relevant technical jargon. The following brief list of terms is for readers who wish to pursue these topics further in the readings listed below: *attitude change, attribution theory, cognitive dissonance theory* (including the *effort justification hypothesis* and *reactance*) as well as other theories of *cognitive consistency,* the *halo effect,* the *Hawthorne effect,* and *role theory* (including the theory of *reference groups*). Other topics in social psychology are better treated by references in the above clinical psychology section. Barber's book on hypnosis deals with the effects of *demand characteristics, expectancy,* and *suggestion.* Similarly, Ullmann and Krasner's book on behavior modification deals with *labeling, modeling,* the *sick role,* and *social learning*

159

theory. The books on communications theory deal extensively with *double bind theory* (or the theory of *paradoxical communications*).

GENERAL

JONES, E. J., AND GERARD, H. B. *Foundations of Social Psychology.* New York: Wiley, 1969.

KRECH, D., CRUTCHFIELD, R. S., AND BALLACHEY, E. L. *Individual in Society.* New York: McGraw-Hill, 1962.

These are both social psychology textbooks. *Foundations of Social Psychology* is newer and contains references to more recent developments in the field. It is much more restricted in scope, focusing on experimental (as opposed to correlational) studies, and it requires more background in psychology from its readers. *Individual in Society,* by contrast, is often used as a text for undergraduate social psychology courses. Although less rigorous and less difficult than the other book, it deals with issues such as mass communications, society, and culture which are almost entirely absent from *Foundations of Social Psychology.*

DEUTSCH, M., AND KRAUSS, R. M. *Theories in Social Psychology.* New York: Basic Books, 1965.

This brief and clear book is an excellent introduction to the major theories of social psychology.

GOFFMAN, E. *The Presentation of Self in Everyday Life.* Garden City, N. Y.: Doubleday Anchor Books, 1959.

Erving Goffman is a skilled observer of behavior, and this book contains an illuminating discussion of social behavior in terms of role theory. Goffman's discussion has obvious implications for understanding why a therapist and a patient perform for each other as they do.

160

Annotated Bibliography

GROUPS

SCHUTZ, W. C. *Joy: Expanding Human Awareness*. New York: Grove Press, 1967.
GUNTHER, B. *Sense Relaxation: Below Your Mind*. New York: Collier Books, 1968.
YABLONSKY, L. *The Tunnel Back: Synanon*. New York: Macmillan, 1965.

Joy and *Sense Relaxation* are two of the best known books of the "touchie-feelie" variety. They contain a plethora of healing rituals—or experiments in being alive, depending on your point of view. *The Tunnel Back* is the fascinating, though by now slightly dated, account of the origin of Synanon and the way of life of its members. The book contains a vivid description of the Synanon Game (then called the small-"s" synanon), which provides an interesting contrast to the approach of the other two books. None of the three books presumes a background in academic psychology.

Ethical Issues

SZASZ, T. S. *The Myth of Mental Illness: Foundations of a Theory of Personal Conduct*. New York: Hoeber-Harper, 1961.

In this, his best known book, as in his other writings, Thomas Szasz argues that the term *mental illness* refers not to an illness but to problems in living and that people who are labeled mentally ill often suffer disastrously as a result.

GOFFMAN, E. *Asylums: Essays on the Social Situation of Mental Patients and Other Inmates*. New York: Doubleday Anchor Books, 1961.

In this book, Erving Goffman directs his keen eye to the life of patients in mental hospitals. He makes it clear that patients' "bizarre" behavior is primarily an adjustment to the institution they must live in rather than a symptom of their illness.

Index

Index

164